NURSING
DOCUMENTATION

NURSING DOCUMENTATION

Legal Focus Across Practice Settings

Sue E. Meiner

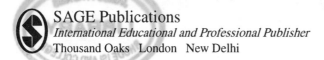

SAGE Publications
International Educational and Professional Publisher
Thousand Oaks   London   New Delhi

Copyright © 1999 by Sage Publications, Inc.

For information:

SAGE Publications, Inc.
2455 Teller Road
Thousand Oaks, California 91320
E-mail: order@sagepub.com

SAGE Publications Ltd.
6 Bonhill Street
London EC2A 4PU
United Kingdom

SAGE Publications India Pvt. Ltd.
M-32 Market
Greater Kailash I
New Delhi 110048 India

Printed in the United States of America

Library of Congress Cataloging-in-Publication Data

Nursing documentation: Legal focus across practice settings/ Sue E. Meiner.
  p. cm.
  Includes bibliographical references and index.
  ISBN 0-7619-1071-9 (cloth: alk. paper).—ISBN 0-7619-1072-7 (paper:
alk. paper)
  1. Nursing records—Miscellanea—Handbooks, manuals, etc.
  2. Nursing—Law and legislation—Handbooks, manuals, etc.
  3. Communication in nursing—Miscellanea—Handbooks, manuals, etc.
  4. Liability, Legal—Miscellanea—Handbooks, manuals, etc.
  I. Meiner, Sue E.
  [DNLM: 1. Nursing Records—legislation & jurisprudence—United
States. 2. Liability, Legal—United States. 3. Risk Management.
  4. Communication. WY 33 AA1 N974 1999]
  RT50.N87 1999
  610.73—dc21
  DNLM/DLC   99-10239

99 00 01 02 03 04 8 7 6 5 4 3 2 1

Acquiring Editor:	Dan Ruth
Production Editor:	Wendy Westgate
Editorial Assistant:	Nevair Kabakian
Typesetter/Designer:	Danielle Dillahunt
Indexer:	Molly Hall
Cover Designer:	Kristi White

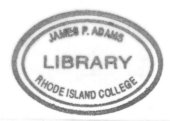

Contents

List of Tables,
Examples, and Charts

Preface

During the past decade, the need to increase instruction regarding legal aspects of nursing has grown dramatically. Traditionally, survey courses with names like "Professional Relationships" or "Legal Aspects of Nursing" were limited to discussions of states' nurse practice acts and basic reviews of nursing negligence, because nurses were employed primarily in acute care institutions that used simple narrative style in nurses' notes to describe care. The recent expansion of nursing in terms of practice settings and scope of practice is demanding of nurses a greater understanding of this aspect of patient care, which in turn has required more extensive instruction on legal implications of charting, reporting, and communicating in the nursing curriculum.

Fueling this need is the enhanced complexity of the professional nurse's role. Medical-surgical nurses now operate primarily in critical care units. Emergency nurses have taken on increased responsibilities in trauma care, minor surgery care, and triage. Obstetric nursing is now almost exclusively a high-risk practice, becoming a fertile ground for litigation when an unfavorable birth outcome occurs. Pediatric nurses have seen an increase in the numbers of physical and substance abuse issues involving family members. The shift to home health care has dramatically increased the extent to which nurses are performing subacute skills in the home. Psychiatric/mental health nursing has moved from institutional to outpatient settings with home care components. All of these changes have placed nurses at great risk of litigation.

For advanced practice nurses, the potential legal exposure is even greater and is compounded by a relative dearth of information on legal issues and risk avoidance. Recent changes in legislation have enabled advanced practice nurses—be they clinical nurse specialists or nurse practitioners—to practice autonomously under an assigned primary provider code. Legal pitfalls proliferate in long-term and extended care facilities, where nurse administrators must grapple with the considerable federal information requirements, each carrying its share of risk. Hazards exist even for nurse educators, as litigation is no longer unheard of in academic settings. Students have legal expectations and obligations that often are omitted from instructor orientation and even nurse education curricula.

The recognition of these myriad issues and the absence of a comprehensive source to address them led to the development of *Nursing Documentation: Legal Focus Across Practice Settings.* The objective was daunting: to attempt to provide a text-reference for individual nurses, nursing education programs at all levels, and clinical and administrative units across the spectrum of health care. Although I believe that these are the audiences who will gain most from the book, it may also benefit physicians and physicians' office staff, insurance companies, law firms and law schools, medical records departments, and in general, any clinical practice site.

The four major parts of the book were developed to be read independently, although generally, the content moves from general information on record keeping systems and general reporting and recording of health care communications, to an overview of legalities and rules surrounding nursing practice and the health care arena, and thence to specific nursing practice settings. The final part of the book presents a dialogue anticipating problems and concerns involving computer database health care records. When appropriate, some of the chapters are followed by case studies chosen from hundreds of case law records. Where changes were made in case law, newer cases were selected. As in any dynamic profession, case law is being created every court day. The reader is encouraged to keep abreast of the changes in the law as they pertain to medical malpractice and the nurse practice acts that are applicable to practitioners of health care in each state.

The writing of any work of this length is a fearsome undertaking not without obstacles and challenges, and this book is no exception. I do believe that it can serve as an asset to practice, however, and I hope you gain as much from reading it as I have gained from creating it.

—Sue E. Meiner, Ed.D., R.N., C.S., G.N.P.

Primum Non Nocere.

First, do no harm.

Acknowledgments

Acknowledging and thanking the professionals who had input into this book is a pleasure. The contributors included registered nurses experienced in a variety of practice settings. This range of talent assisted in making each chapter more applicable to the broad spectrum of nursing practice. To the many friends who never tired of answering questions about specifics in the various practice areas included in this book, a heartfelt thanks seems too little an acknowledgment.

I gratefully acknowledge Alice Rini, a registered nurse and practicing attorney, who devoted time and energy into the writing of chapters that required a thorough knowledge of the law and health care.

A special thanks goes to Betsy Mueth for her cheerleading along the way and her assistance with obtaining current reference materials. As a nursing college librarian, she provided knowledge and assistance in the computer-based medical records and in current nursing applications.

There are many other behind-the-scenes contributors to the production of this book. Daniel Ruth, an editor at Sage Publications, encouraged the development of this book while staying the course during rough weather. Wendy Westgate, the production editor on this book, was a pleasure to work with—I appreciated her professionalism combined with constant good humor. Anna Howland, an editorial assistant at Sage and a consummate organizer, scrutinized the manuscript before production. Appreciation goes to the many production professionals at Sage. Special thanks go to the copy editor and the indexer, without whose attention to details, addenda or errata might have been needed.

This project could not have been done without the total support and encouragement of family and friends. I especially thank a very special person in my life who provided absolute support during the months of research, writing, and rewriting. To Robert Edward Meiner, my husband and best friend for the past three decades, a very special appreciation is extended. He faithfully prepared meals and late-night snacks, made middle-of-the-night trips to the copy center, screened phone calls endlessly, and did not complain when vacations were eliminated during the writing process.

To one and all, thank you so very much.

PART 1

COMMUNICATIONS IN NURSING PRACTICE

INTRODUCTION TO DOCUMENTATION, LIABILITY, AND NURSING PRACTICE

1

Sue E. Meiner

Chapter Outline

The past decade of advances in medical care and technology has led to multiple changes in health care delivery systems and third-party payment practices. Other dramatic changes have included the public's awareness for a need to learn as much as possible about medical care to make informed decisions. The increasing communications technology within the United States and in other Western countries has informed, alarmed, complicated, and in some ways created skepticism toward the health care providers and insurance companies. This dynamic alteration in the role of the American health care system has created a risk of increased liability for all health care workers.

Nursing negligence has been given little publicity while the news media frequently report physician and hospital malpractice claims. The overwhelming majority of all malpractice events happen in acute care settings and often involve one or more nurses along with the physician of record. The cause for many claims can be attributed to errors made by the nursing staff. At the heart of litigation is the medical record. The purpose of this book is to enhance awareness of the need to improve nursing documentation as a component of written communication among health care workers, including physicians. A major benefit will be to reduce litigation based on faulty or omitted recording and reporting of patient care data in the medical record.

Nurses have an integral relationship among all members of the health care team and the recipients of their care. While delivering nursing care to patients, nurses have responsibilities that include meeting standards of care delineated by law, national nursing organizations, and public expectations. Other responsibilities are to provide cost-effective care delivery. Cost-effectiveness of health care is a necessity that encompasses the health care system as an employer, the third-party reimbursement system, and the cost to the patient. Long-term costs may include salary issues and even the viability of some health care delivery systems.

In this complex climate, litigation has increased in number, scope, and monetary awards to the plaintiffs. The number of malpractice or nursing negligence claims has increased in proportion to the settlement figures. When hospitals, extended care facilities, or nursing homes are named in legal actions, nurses more frequently are included in the broad namings of responsible parties to claims of malpractice. Nurses are responsible for the care that they administer. They also are responsible for having sufficient knowledge concerning health care delivery to be able to identify mistakes of some other members of the health care team, prior to actions that could adversely affect the patient's care. When mistakes or incomplete/unclear orders by physicians are not identified and/or corrected by the nursing staff, the potential for patient injury intensifies.

An astute nurse acting as a patient advocate can remedy a potential error in treatment through swift and decisive action. The nurse no longer is in a servant role to the physician but, rather, is a complementary health care provider working in concert with the physician for the patient's best outcome. As such, the nurse should strive to understand the basis for frequently encountered patient care situations. In the late 1990s, the registered nurse's (RN) educational preparation includes using critical judgments to analyze new situations and make appropriate patient care decisions.

Nurses have gained the role of making independent judgments and actions regarding patient care. At the same time, this responsibility has increased the risk of liability. The impact of additional regulations from licensing boards and the results of court cases has altered the relationships of nursing to society. As the practice of practical, professional, and advanced practice nursing has dynamically developed, more emphasis is being placed on documentation of nursing actions.

COMMUNICATIONS IN NURSING PRACTICE

Chapter 2 introduces the variety of records and reports that make up the system of health care documentation. Former documentation systems included only narrative nurses notes within a handwritten medical record. Other forms of handwritten records developed over the past three decades include the problem-intervention-evaluation (PIE), subjective-objective-assessment-plan (SOAP), and problem-oriented medical record (POMR) formats. Some facilities use outcome-based charting and/or charting by exception formats. With the use of critical paths, different documentation concerns are being recognized.

These handwritten records are maintained within a reasonable distance from the point of health care delivery. In an acute care setting, these records frequently are kept at a main reporting area (nurses station) or in the patient's room/unit cabinet. In a primary care setting, the patient's file normally is placed in a medical record room or filing area within the office when not in active use (Iyer and Camp, 1995).

Chapter 3 will discuss the current and developing computerized record systems. The increased uses of computers in the workforce have given rise to computerized medical records, computerized data retrieval systems, and bedside computer data entry systems. With this expansion of the use of computers in record keeping, trends in documentation have undergone continuous alterations.

As computerized medical records continue to proliferate, the liability issues of documentation become clouded with concerns of timeliness, inadvertent breach of confidentiality, and importance of careful and complete documentation at the time of service or care. Methods for changing information charted by mistake and issues of late data entry will pose special problems for the computerized medical record (Milholland and Heiler, 1996).

Different nursing service areas have different recording methods and standards for documentation. Hospital or acute care settings have had strict regulations for the management of medical records through the state licensing boards and the Joint Commission on Accreditation of Healthcare Organizations (JCAHO, 1996). Long-term/extended care facilities and nursing homes are even more strictly regulated by state agencies for the aging and/or people with disabilities as well as by Medicare and JCAHO. Home health care, community health centers, ambulatory clinics, physicians' offices, and other sites for health care delivery have a mosaic of rules, regulations, and patterns of documentation and maintenance of medical records. This further complicates the understanding of the standards of care in relation to maintaining complete, understandable, and protected medical records that are quite different in different practice settings.

Failure to communicate with other members of the health care team when abnormal findings or occurrences develop is another area of liability that will be presented in Chapter 4. Knowing about abnormal events without reporting or recording them can lead to claims of nursing negligence. Every patient expects to receive competent nursing care in a multitude of dimensions including reporting and recording of the events that occurred during the period of time in which care was being provided.

Documentation must include information related to events that require reporting or relaying information to other members of the health care team. Chapters 5 and 6 will provide information related to observation reporting,

TABLE 1.1 Components of a Contract

1. Consent by both parties (nurse and employer, nurse and patient, nurse and physician, nurse and family, or nurse and community)
2. Service of value being exchanged
3. Purpose for the contract
4. Parties involved are competent to make the agreement
5. A legally appropriate contract form is used

contacts with other health care providers and family members, and reporting of abnormal situations encountered in health care practices.

LEGAL FOCUS ON NURSING COMMUNICATIONS AND DOCUMENTATION

The performance of licensed nursing at any level involves an agreement for the exchange of services within a contract. This is quite different from moral agreements or social obligation agreements that are not classified as contracts. Contracts are enforceable by law, and the components that must be met are listed in Table 1.1. When a contract is broken, compensation can be awarded as a remedy to the person or estate of the party claiming to have suffered by the breach (Guido, 1997; Trandel-Korenchuk and Trandel-Korenchuk, 1997).

The nurse-patient relationship is at the heart of nursing care. Whenever a nurse renders services to a patient, a legal relationship (contract) begins. Once this relationship exists, legal consequences of all actions of the nurse are open for examination by standards of care. These standards follow a basic underpinning of actions that analyze the specific care given by examining what another reasonable and prudent nurse with similar education would do in a like situation.

Understanding nurses' rights, legal status, and liability issues is an essential step to safely conduct the practice of nursing skills. Although contracts confer a legal relationship, liability for negligent acts does not depend solely on a legal contract or relationship between the nurse and another party. Negligent acts are not dismissed for services that are given gratuitously. In some states, when an injury occurs to a patient while being cared for by a nurse, a lawsuit for damages can be brought by that patient or by concerned others.

Humanitarian obligations often place nurses in active roles during emergency events. During an emergency situation, a nurse is considered to be responsible for actions that exemplify the education, training, and skills of a similar nurse. Actions taken rarely are considered to be similar to those of the medically unskilled. The performance of any medical act that will preserve life or limb usually is exempt from liability. The key is the term *emergency action*.

Care must be given when actions are taken beyond the scope of practice or licensure in situations that are not truly life-or-death emergencies (Bernzweig, 1996).

"Good Samaritan" legislation is designed to allow health care providers to offer first aid in emergency situations while providing protection from malpractice suits. Although many states subscribe to this special protection, some do not permit any leeway in the responsibility of licensed nurses providing emergency care to persons where no special duty exists. Therefore, the voluntary performance of nursing skills in emergency situations becomes an ethical issue instead of a purely legal one. Some states and Canada have taken the "duty to rescue" into a compulsory level. Minnesota and Vermont have statutory laws that require health care professionals to provide aid to victims of grave physical harm or when lives are in peril. Failure to render medical assistance can result in charges, ranging from petty misdemeanor to a criminal offense. Most Canadian provinces have enacted compulsory assistance statutes that require all persons to give aid to others when the need arises (Guido, 1997, p. 103).

Nursing Negligence

Chapter 7 will present information that is basic to understanding legal principles appropriate to nursing liability. The legal principles inherent in standards of care have become a major issue in nursing negligence cases.

Legal principles that have a direct bearing on nursing actions after the fact are not always clearly identified. Identifying the actions of a reasonably prudent nurse usually is found in the documentation of nursing actions in the medical record.

Consent for treatment is another area that can become a legal issue for nursing care. Establishing consent for treatment might seem as simple as approaching a patient and beginning to administer a treatment or medication. However, this routine action by nurses needs prior consideration to avoid the potential of battery (Quigley, 1991a, 1991b).

Another topic of basic information concerns the time limits imposed on medical negligence claims. It is the statute of limitations that provides a finite time frame to most incidents that could possibly result in legal claims. However, many exceptions to this statute exist.

Risk Management

The functions of the risk management unit within an acute care facility are less often understood by health care personnel. As a result, it might be seen as a group of punitive individuals who ask questions placing staff members in defensive stances. The requests made by risk management are seen as taking time away from patient care. Chapter 8 will present information related to risk management. Common causes and the prevention of specific malpractice claims, as they relate to communication and documentation topics, will be discussed. Issues of claims management and continuous quality improvement programs to reduce the risk of liability will be overviewed. Reviewing this information should assist in reducing the unknown factor that causes stress among health care workers.

DOCUMENTATION IN PRACTICE SETTINGS

The role of the staff nurse employed in an acute care facility has changed immeasurably over the past decade. Patients are much sicker, stay in the facility fewer days or even for just hours, and frequently are transferred to different units during a single short stay. Establishing a therapeutic nurse-patient relationship after a few brief contacts with the patient is difficult for many nurses. The rapid turnover of patients has created nursing care planning that has less chance of being fully accomplished within the too-brief patient contact period.

The act of planning for the patient's discharge on admission was initiated in the late 1980s. Unless an admission is an emergency, patient information is available, prior to admission, from prescreening calls by hospital personnel or from physicians' office records. Currently, this information initiates the discharge planning prior to admission. Changes in discharge options require the attention of the case manager in most acute care settings. Although the bedside nurse has input into the proposed continuation of care following discharge, the end decision is one made by the third-party payment company. Many times, the plan presented by the nurse is not approved for implementation by a representative of the health care delivery system.

Documentation becomes a vital link in presenting the true picture of a patient's condition. If the failure to approve the plan is based on omissions of needed information related to specific nursing care needs at home after discharge, then the patient's record can be resubmitted to the case manager for additional review before a final decision is rendered. As is evident, documentation becomes an essential tool for continuity of adequate patient care.

Staffing and Delegation Issues

As nurses are being moved from nursing units of familiarity to those of convenience, special needs and issues arise. Accepting patient care assignments in unfamiliar nursing specialties, such as emergency departments, obstetrical units, psychiatry, pediatrics, or postanesthesia areas, can prove disastrous for unprepared nurses. Changes in practice behaviors of nurses, related to patient assignments, are becoming more commonplace. Whereas the past practice behaviors were to accept any patient assignment, the current trend is to refuse an assignment based on personal nursing liability issues. The most frequently recognized cause for assignment refusal is the lack of skills or experience in an unfamiliar setting. Not all assignments can be refused. When this case exists, some facilities use a formal document called "Assignment Despite Objection." This completed form can be submitted to nursing management to provide a statement in the record in the event of an untoward patient occurrence with injury (Missouri Nurses Association, 1996). This might serve as an alert to a pending problem for nursing management.

Chapter 9 will discuss staffing issues concerning the unanticipated moving of staff nurses, licensed practical/vocational nurses, or unlicensed assistive personnel to a unit where different skills are required from those on the home unit. When nurses are "floated" to or "pulled" from customary nursing care units, delegation issues can become risky for the charge nurse or nurse manager on the receiving end (Huber, 1996).

Supervision and delegation issues also are safety issues for the patient. The delegating process has murky areas that need to be addressed, especially because of the increase in hiring nurse extenders or unlicensed assistive personnel instead of retaining an all-RN patient care staff (Ketter, 1994). Chapter 9 also will discuss supervision and delegation issues.

Specialty Nursing Units

The complexities of the higher specialized areas within an acute care facility call for alertness in the unique needs for documentation of that specialty. Charting methods for nursing practice differ within specialty areas of acute care nursing. The areas that will be addressed in Chapters 10 through 15 are emergency departments, critical care units, obstetrics, pediatrics, perioperative nursing, and psychiatric/mental health nursing, respectively. When documentation records for special units are being created or revised, special attention to the unique needs of patients and the services required is essential to establish relevant written communication tools. The standards of care will be measured by the thoroughness and accuracy of these records (Branson, 1996; Fairchild, 1993; Urden, Davie, and Thelan, 1992).

Community and Home Nursing

Community nursing and home care nursing have proliferated from the advent of the federally mandated diagnosis-related groupings (DRGs) in the 1980s. The reduced length of stay in acute care settings led to the need for subacute or continued care outside of hospitals. Following implementation of DRGs, Medicare-certified home health care agencies grew from less than 2,000 nationally to an estimated 9,000-plus currently. In 1996, the National Association for Home Care reported 8,747 agencies.

In Chapter 16, attention will be given to home care nursing. Documentation is a means of communication among the home visiting nurse and the nursing supervisor at the agency's office, the physician, and other allied health care providers. Recording is a time-consuming task for the home care nurse. The record reflects all interactions in the home with patients and family, teaching and training, and direct care. Contact with the physician always should be documented, even if done so with brevity.

The teaching and training issues are vital in home care. Indication of exact information given to the patient and family members for them to properly monitor the condition must be made in written form. Information on reporting concerns or emergencies must be charted, and similar information must be made available in the home for the caregivers' use, if necessary. Recording all of the information that is required may be done in writing, by dictation using a handheld model, or by using a laptop or notebook computer.

With any method, timing is important. Charting should be done as soon as possible following the care rendered. Transcription of dictated nurses notes also should be done as soon as possible following the care rendered. This usually is done by a transcriptionist at the main office and is ready for review and signature within a reasonable amount of time, as determined by agency policy.

Extended and Long-Term Care

The residents of extended and long-term care facilities usually are dependent on the care and concern demonstrated by bedside caregivers. Because so many of the individuals residing in these facilities are not able to care for their own personal daily activity needs, nursing has the important role of providing safe care that directly relates to the specific needs of individual residents. As their needs change, the nursing care plan also must change. To ensure that the most chronically ill citizens of the United States are given appropriate care, several mechanisms for documentation have evolved.

Chapter 17 will present extended and long-term care documentation issues that have developed into a maze of paperwork. Abbreviations such as "MDS 2.0" and "RAP" are well known as time-consuming but required forms of documentation. The minimum data set (MDS) and the resident assessment protocol (RAP) standardize information that validates compliance with quality improvement and provides the foundation for the resident's plan of care. The turnover of patients in these facilities is not as rapid as in the acute care setting, but the time frame for completion of these lengthy and quite detailed documents is set by standards. Therefore, documentation is critical to the admission of a patient and can be very costly if deficiencies are found during a survey process. The federal government, under the supervision of the Health Care Financing Administration (HCFA), oversees compliance issues in long-term care facilities/nursing homes. Civil and monetary penalties can be assessed for noncompliance (HCFA, 1994).

Advanced Practice Nursing

Nursing practice has expanded into areas that previously were restricted to medical practice. This expansion of responsibilities and services has increased the risk of malpractice. Examples of failure to meet the standards of care include a failure to refer a patient to a medical doctor in a timely manner and a failure to order or interpret diagnostic services or treatments, which can lead to a decline in health, further injury, disability, or death. An added standard of care is applied to an advanced practice nurse (APN) in the performance of duties associated with the responsibilities of specific certified specialties. This is due to the additional education and training beyond the basic licensure requirements and the results of passing a national certification examination validating the advanced knowledge and status.

Chapter 18 will continue with information related to the APN. The disclosure of limitations in treatment options, when primary care is rendered by an advanced practice nurse/nurse practitioner (APN/NP), is a duty of that health care provider. When an illness is beyond the scope of practice of the APN/NP, a referral is expected to be made to a physician or specialist. Failure to do so might provide a foundation for liability and will place the practice of the expanded role of the APN/NP in a precarious position with licensing agencies.

Nursing Education

Nursing education and administration might seem to be distant to documentation scrutiny toward potential litigation. The fact is that individuals entering into a nursing education program come for different reasons. In previous decades, nursing students were drawn to the field by a desire to nurture and care for the sick and injured. Monetary and benefit issues were given secondary consideration over the actual job placement in a hospital. The altruistic nature of nursing no longer predominates.

Women and men in the late 1990s enter the field of nursing for vastly different purposes than did nursing students of several decades ago. Career mobility might mean that a nursing student does not plan on giving direct physical care to patients but, rather, plans on moving rapidly up a corporate ladder or laterally into a non-patient care nursing position. Nursing educators with many years of experience continue to consider attitude toward the profession as an important element to providing quality nursing care to patients. With the exception of a category called professionalism, the measurement of attitude frequently is seen as too subjective to be evaluated "fairly." In some university programs, the measurement of attitude has been removed from the evaluative process of student performance. This has led to the passing of clinical courses and ultimately graduating students with less than desirable personality and communication attributes for delivering personal care to individuals.

Chapter 19 will look at documentation of the curriculum, faculty records, student records, and contracts for clinical placement of students. These are among the many records reviewed by licensing and accreditation agencies. Colleges of nursing also are reviewed by regional collegiate accreditation bodies. The documentation fills an entire room for the time that these groups of examiners are present. Complete, comprehensive, and accurate record keeping and documentation is essential for licensing and accreditation for nursing programs.

Following the academic process, students become graduates. This new role creates challenges that must be given appropriate attention.

After graduation and successful completion of the national examination for licensure, nurses need to practice learned ways of documenting patient assessments, plans for care, treatments and responses, medications and reactions, and communication with other significant individuals. Careful transfer of information from physician orders as well as pharmacy, dietary, and other departments within an acute care setting is essential. Nurses will expand documentation techniques by working on methods and formats that will deliver the most comprehensive information in the smallest space. Gaps in the medical record are a major reason for malpractice litigation against health care providers.

Nurses who select to work outside of acute care settings will need to take courses or in-service classes on the specifics of nursing documentation for that arena of practice. Whenever new systems of documentation are being developed, nurses need to insist on being a part of that innovative team and not fall back in complacency while letting others create a product that might not meet the true needs of the practice setting. Nursing educators and educational administrators are committed to a continuous focus on documentation intricacies in the multifaceted arena of nursing preparation.

Managed Care and Nursing

Chapter 20 will provide a brief glimpse into managed care and the nursing role. Documentation of the nurse's professional endeavors will be discussed in relation to the credentialing and privileging process.

Managed care was formed as a health care delivery system that offered cost-effective services for subscribers at reduced or constant rates. Since the inception of this delivery system, a continuously changing concept of the form of managed care has evolved.

Managed care aimed at reducing national health care expenditures through elimination of duplication of services by curtailing unnecessary diagnostic tests and procedures as practiced for defense protection from litigation. The system that evolved is complex, confusing, and often viewed as limiting needed and life-saving therapy and surgical procedures.

CONCLUSION

As the current health care delivery system continues to diversify, documentation of the actual care delivered to patients becomes more critical. Litigation in areas of malpractice continues to increase, as do the monetary awards being given by the jury system. Nurses are being added to litigation, if not singled out for naming in negligence cases. Medical records are a means to communicate with other health care team members and to provide a written record of the care given to a patient. Nursing documentation must reflect current standards of nursing practice that are individualized for a specific patient. The record needs to reflect the patient's needs, problems, limitations, and reactions to the nursing interventions implemented following identification of nursing diagnoses. Thus, the goal-directed nursing care that is provided following the nursing process should be able to be easily identified in the documentation of the medical record.

CURRENT APPROACHES IN CHARTING 2

Sue E. Meiner

Chapter Outline

The traditional paper and chart medical record has been the stable form of charting of patient care throughout nursing's long history beginning with Florence Nightingale. As computer technology has permeated everyday business, the medical record has slowly shifted from the paper-based system to one of computer-based records (CBRs). This chapter discusses charting that originally was intended for the paper and chart medical record. The formats discussed are focus charting (FOCUS), charting by exception (CBE), problem-intervention-evaluation (PIE), subjective-objective-assessment-plan (SOAP), and the problem-oriented medical record (POMR). Content on outcome-based charting and narrative nurses notes is included. Chapter 3 will discuss the newest trends and concerns with the CBR.

During the past 25 years, nursing charting has continuously taken on an increasingly important role in recording care given to a patient and the response of the patient to that care. Three elements have been instrumental in the increasing role and responsibility for thorough charting: changes in nursing practice and responsibility, regulatory agency requirements, and the legal environment in which guidelines reflect the standard of care.

The general public has expectations of the care given by nurses to be effective and of high quality. The evidence of the care given by nurses must be charted in the medical record and be available to the patient or an attorney for scrutiny. The attorney views the patient's medical record as evidence of the care and health management given. When the chart is reviewed and found to contain essential information that is accurate, carefully done, and complete, litigation may be avoided.

DOCUMENTING THE NURSING PROCESS

Elements within the Nurse Practice Act of each state discuss using and documenting the nursing process when providing nursing care to patients and charting the care given. Specifically mentioned in most state statutes is the use of nursing diagnosis, planning, and interventions with outcome evaluation that follows the patient assessment and data collection. With the inclusion of the nursing process in the practice act, nurses are legally bound to use this systematic method for patient care. The Joint Commission on Accreditation of Healthcare Organizations (JCAHO) reaffirms the emphasis of using the nursing process regardless of the charting method selected by the individual facility. Problem-or source-oriented recording formats must reflect the use of the nursing process as well. The use of the nursing process in charting follows the scientific method of problem solving within a health care environment (Iyer and Camp, 1995; Kerr, 1992).

The specific elements of the nursing process include assessment (physical and other data collection), nursing diagnosis (North American Nursing Diagnosis Association [NANDA]), planning (nursing care plan), implementing (nursing interventions), and evaluating services and care delivered (ongoing or outcome based). When charting follows the steps of the nursing process, a thorough picture evolves with the following components:

1. Factual information
2. Accurate and reliable
3. Complete details
4. Brief and concise
5. Timely with current data
6. Logical organization of material

According to Potter and Perry (1995), "The record should explain measures needed for continuity and consistency of care" (p. 184). Charting should include the nurse's judgment and evaluation of care and the patient's condition. Each area of the nursing process adds to the total picture of the ongoing management of care within the delivery system. "The record provides data that nurses use to identify and support nursing diagnoses and plan proper interventions for care" (p. 184).

When charting the nursing process, the initial step of *assessment* needs to contain information from the patient, family members, and/or significant others. The health assessment is derived from the health history, physical examination, diagnostic test results, and review of previous health records (when available). In many institutions, old medical records are delivered to the acute care nursing unit for review by the physician and the nursing caregivers.

Following the analysis of information, a nursing diagnosis is formulated based on available data and nursing judgments. The planning phase includes prioritizing care by the level of importance to the health status of the patient. This phase must keep outcome criteria based on mutual goals set by the interaction of the nurse and patient. All outcome criteria must have a time line with target dates that indicate intervention evaluation. The intervention or implementation pertains to the actual performance of the plan of care.

Objective data analysis is used to determine the success or failure of the outcome of care. When the outcome is found to be in deficit according to preplanned goals, reassessment is begun again and the cycle of the nursing process is reinstituted (Springhouse, 1995).

FOCUS CHARTING

Using nursing diagnosis as the focus of an entry into the nursing progress notes, the elements of FOCUS take shape. Charting is directed at patient-centered problems. A four-column page is divided into small columns for date and time, a slightly larger column for stating the nursing diagnosis (labeled the "focus" column), and a column greater than half of the width of the page for the progress notes. The code for writing progress notes is the acronym DAR, where D is data, A is action, and R is response. Data are written with subjective and objective information. Action can include statements related to current and future nursing interventions as well as plan of care changes due to assessment findings. Response is related to the patient's reactions to any health care interventions.

Although most recording is directly related to a nursing diagnosis, the focus column can include other issues rather than a nursing diagnosis. An example of another issue could be visits made by other health-care or non-health-care disciplines, with patient responses recorded before and after the visits. This format requires the use of multiple pages of flow sheets, instructional classes for new employees, and review to discourage using the progress notes as a narrative statement of care (Springhouse, 1995). Table 2.1 provides a sample of FOCUS.

CHARTING BY EXCEPTION

This system of recording assessments, interventions, and responses was developed to eliminate redundancy and to organize information in a manner that would reduce errors in charting. When used following a thorough orientation to the guidelines and protocols established for nursing assessment and interventions, CBE can save time, reduce repetition of charting, and provide immediate identification of significant changes in a patient's condition. However, in the presence of unclear nursing guidelines or lacking other flow sheets that are needed for recording other care or treatments, CBE can open legal interpretation

TABLE 2.1 Sample of FOCUS Charting

[plate stamp here] Patient I.D.: Wills, Mary Dr. Karl: Adm 52200 320 North Hall Bed 2 SS#: 123-45-6789			Hospital #: 123456a

DATE	TIME	FOCUS/NURSING DIAGNOSIS	NURSING PROGRESS NOTES
5/22/00	0900	Altered Comfort	D: requested pain medication for post-op incisional discomfort, 7 on a 1-10 scale.
			A: Demerol 75mg, IM, LUOQ, repositioned, side rails up, instructed to call for assistance
	0935		R: States she feels much better and the pain is a 2 on a 1-10 scale. —Vivi Able, RN

of a breach in standards of nursing care. The evaluation of nursing interventions can be difficult to identify if the records are confusing or incomplete (Burke and Murphy, 1995).

Unlike in FOCUS, the progress notes in CBE are used to document revisions to the plan of care and other interventions that do not fit the guidelines for recording on the nursing medical order flow sheet. Therefore, the progress notes rarely contain any information related to assessments or interventions.

The main recording form is the nursing medical order flow sheet. This 24-hour flow sheet uses specific key abbreviations that must be used consistently for accuracy. Although this single form is the usual finding in a chart system using CBE, some facilities combine different data on the same form as the nursing medical order flow sheet. Recording hygiene measures lends itself well to a flow sheet format in CBE. If the standard care is given, then notations are not needed. A check mark is the only identification of completion of routine hygiene care.

Tammelleo (1994) discussed the difficulties that CBE was experiencing. The report noted that hospitals had been found liable for claims of breach of standards of care when discernible understandings of patients' conditions or outcomes of care were problematic.

TABLE 2.2 Basic Sample of Charting by Exception Form

PATIENT ASSESSMENT AND PROGRESS NOTES

DATE _____
TIME _____   INITIAL ASSESSMENT   DATE/TIME

CONSCIOUSNESS:		
ORIENTATION:		
PUPILS:		
MOVEMENT:		
HEART RATE: RHYTHM: Reg. or Irreg.		
VASCULAR CHECKS:		
SKIN:		
EDEMA:		
IV: SITE:		
DSG △: _____		
RESP. RATE:		
COUGH / SPUTUM:		
TREATMENTS:		
FOLEY:		
VOID:		
BOWEL SOUNDS: BM _____		
DIET _____		
FEED: ASSIST / TOTAL: APPETITE_____		
TUBE FEEDING:		

TYPE: DRAINAGE:
1.
2.
3.
4.
5.

LOCATION	APPEARANCE	TREATMENT

LOCATION	TYPE	RESPONSE TO TREATMENT

SIGNATURE

HYGIENE	ACTIVITY	SIDE RAILS	SAFETY	LABS TEST / PROCEDURES

On the pro-CBE side, Burke and Murphy (1995) upheld their previous stance that if all standards are met, only the exceptions to the norm need to be recorded. They dismissed the premise that if it was not documented it must not have been performed. Table 2.2 provides a sample CBE form.

PIE CHARTING

This form of charting is not inclusive of all the information necessary to document the entire nursing process. However, it was developed from a nursing perspective and basics of the nursing process in 1984 at Craven County Hospital in New Bern, North Carolina. The acronym of PIE stands for *problem* presented

TABLE 2.3 Sample of PIE Charting

Patient I.D.: Doe, Joe 321-54-9876
11/30/29 M Dr. Smith
[plate stamp here] Room 6421 East Tower
Adm # 876543D   Hospital #: 76543

DATE	TIME	NURSING PROBLEM	NURSING NOTES
9/15/00	0800	#2 — Mobility	P.—Mobility, Impaired physical related to decreased strength and endurance secondary to fracture of (L) hip. I.—Maintain body alignment during bedrest. Change position every 2 hours or less while in bed. Encourage shifting position q 30 minutes while in chair. E.—No further impairment of mobility or dependence occurs. Able to be more physically active prior to discharge. Able to explain activity limitations within goals of self care. V. Able RN

(nursing diagnosis), *interventions* (implementation of planned actions), and *evaluation* of the care given (in outcome statements related to the interventions listed). PIE charting does not contain any assessment data per se. The assessment and data collection information is found in another chart form that can vary among settings (Buckley-Womack and Gidney, 1987; Siegrist, Dettor, and Stocks, 1985). Table 2.3 provides a sample of PIE charting.

PROBLEM-ORIENTED MEDICAL RECORD

The nursing process forms the basis for the POMR method of charting patient problems. The foundation of this method is a single list of patient problems generated by members of the health care team. Potter and Perry (1995, p. 187) listed the advantages of this method of charting as follows:

1. Gives emphasis to clients' perceptions of their problems
2. Requires continuous evaluation and revision of care plan
3. Provides greater continuity of care among health care team members
4. Enhances effective communication among health care team members
5. Increases efficiency in gathering data
6. Provides easy-to-read information in chronological order
7. Reinforces use of the nursing process

The chronological problem number is not repeated within the same hospitalization. When the problem is resolved, the list is modified by signing a space or checkoff area next to the listing. The date that the problem was resolved is noted next to the signature. Whereas the POMR list of problems does not contain space for narrative writing, another form is used for anecdotal progress notes identified by the number of the problem from the list. It is this format that can take the form of structured narrative progress notes. The following information pertains to two of the more commonly used formats of structured notes.

SOAP CHARTING

The charting format that is routinely used with the POMR is the method of recording *subjective* information supplied by the patient with *objective* information that is factual and measurable. These data are collected during physical assessments and review of laboratory or diagnostic test results. The *assessment* is developed from nursing judgments determined by the synthesis of the data obtained from the subjective and objective information. The final step in SOAP charting is the *plan*. Immediate short- and long-term measures for resolving the patient's identified problems are reflected in this final step.

As the SOAP format was used, changes evolved that would answer additional questions posed by using the nursing process. Initially, the letter E (for *evaluation*) was added to the acronym. Following the SOAPE format, the letter I (for *intervention*) was added between the plan and evaluation components. The format became the SOAPIE method, allowing an intervention comment to be made. During the process of caregiving, interventions might need to be altered to fully address the patient's problem. The "I" section permitted that change without adding a new or revised problem to the patient's list.

The most current addition to the original SOAP format is the letter R (for *revision*). The acronym for the format becomes SOAPIER. When changes to the original problem come from revised interventions, outcomes of care, or time lines, the "R" section is used to denote that change. This saves renumbering and

TABLE 2.4. Sample of SOAP Charting

Patient I.D.: *Wills, Mary*
Dr. Karl Adam 52200   Hospital #: *123456a*
[plate stamp here] *320 No. Bed 2*
SS# 123-45-6789

DATE	TIME	NURSING PROBLEM	NURSING NOTES
5/24/00	1420	#3	S. – "I am worried that I won't be able to walk to the bathroom when I get home."
			O. – Unsteady gait on walk from bed to bathroom, used the wall for support.
			A. – Strength in both lower extremities is 3/5, H&H wnl, lives alone, has never used a walking aid.
			P. – Physical therapy to begin – strengthening exercises 3X day until discharge, instruct in use of walking aid, obtain author-ization for unit rental if needed, re-evaluate mobility daily and prior to discharge.
			— Veri Able, RN

restating a problem that is essentially the same but with new goals, outcomes, dates, and/or times. Table 2.4 provides a sample of SOAP charting.

These formats are required to be entered into the medical record at least once every 24 hours for each patient problem that is identified in the problem list. Many institutions that currently are using any form of the POMR formats may be adding additional forms to satisfy the full scope of answering the requirements of documenting the nursing process.

NARRATIVE NURSES NOTES

Narrative charting is the most widely understood and used format for charting nursing observations, interventions, and responses to care. The narrative note is a simple technical paragraph headed by the date, time, and information, with the nurse's signature and credentials following each entry. This format includes charting normal assessment findings, routine care, and interventions in detail. The importance of the information often is lost in the length and repetitive writing when narrative nurses notes contain detailed patient care and contact and all activities that have any association with the patient's time during a specific nurse's duty.

After this method of charting became recognized as cumbersome, time-consuming, and repetitive, additional forms were added to the chart in flow sheet style with checkoff boxes in an attempt to reduce the writing time and content. However, this change or addition did not always reduce the narrative notes; in some facilities, it increased the time and writing by the nursing staff. Without proper in-service programs, many nurses continued to write lengthy narrative nurses notes and repeated the same information on flow sheets.

This duplication of information can lead to confusion when the medical record is reviewed by defense or plaintiff attorneys, especially when the records are incomplete in one area of charting and the remainder of the information is in another section of the chart or flow sheet. This also can be looked on as trying to hide or cover up any failures in patient care when the record is not consistent in all areas. The disadvantages of narrative charting are disorganization and task orientation of the notes and that it is time-consuming.

Disorganization is apparent with a lack of structure to the manner in which the information is entered into the narrative format. Task orientation leads to extreme details in every procedure undertaken. A simple dressing change may be recorded in narrative format of more than half a page of nurses notes, depending on the writer's proclivity to maximize detail. The same entry may be repeated word for word every time a repeated dressing change is done. Although the charting of a simple dressing change is not to be considered unimportant, it needs to be written only once, with no further need to go into great detail unless a change in the patient's condition occurs. Table 2.5 provides a sample of narrative nurses notes.

In some cases, the record contains a conflict of information, with opposing statements related to the same data or notations made in different parts of the chart. When this occurs, the charting becomes suspicious and is reviewed for alterations or falsification of the permanent record.

OUTCOME-BASED CHARTING

The process-oriented format of charting frequently is referred to as *outcome-based charting*. The focus of this format is based on patient behavior following nursing interventions. After identifying the patient's problems, formulation of the desired outcomes of the nursing care plan is determined from subjective and

TABLE 2.5. Sample of Narrative Nurses Notes

GENERAL HOSPITAL
1234 Main Street
AnyTown, State

Doe, Jane C. 123-45-7788
10/24/43   M   Dr. Smith
Room 7001   West Wing
Admission # 234156789C

NURSING NOTES

Date	Time	NOTES
2/14/00	1400	Pt. requests PRN pain medication for constant dull ache over the abdominal incision area in right upper quadrant. Rated as a 7 on a scale of 1-10. V.S. 138/88, 92, 18, 37.4°C. No redness or drainage at incisional site, sutures intact, skin well approximated. Able to take 2 oz. ice chips, no nausea or vomiting —V. Able RN
	1405	Demerol 75 mg IM, LUOQ, repositioned, side rails up, instructed to call for assistance —Ver. Able RN
	1435	Resting comfortably, pain reported as a 2 on the same scale of 1-10, repositioned and fresh ice chips given. —V. Able RN

NOTE: do not chart below this line - sign all entries - do not leave blank lines

objective information. With outcome charting, the evaluation process is ongoing throughout the acute care stay.

More recently, critical paths, care paths, and/or care maps have been developed for specific recurring illnesses or operative procedures. A time line is established based on the expected outcomes for a unique identifier (e.g., hysterectomy, myocardial infarction). These forms present a sequential plan of interventions that are to be followed uniformly. When any deviation from the standard care path results, a recognition trigger is activated that requires explanations for the variances. The trigger is not a physical mechanism but, rather, a metaphor for an indicator on the record form. When a trigger is identified, the variance that activated the response will need to be justified or actions taken to correct the problem. If these responses are not acted on, then the variance usually is referred to a care path committee for review of the circumstances that produced an outlier to the established care path. Giuliano and Poirier (1991) found that the use of critical paths avoided any oversights that might compromise patient care and preparation for discharge.

FLOW SHEETS IN CHARTING

When specific repetitive care measures are performed throughout a patient's length of stay in many practice settings, the use of a flow sheet is preferred over the lengthy narrative notes. The flow sheet is designed to contain checkoff boxes that provide for a quick and easy identification of changes in the patient's condition. However, when the flow sheet charting method is used, at times a descriptive narrative note might be needed to further clarify any changes in the patient's condition. The flow sheet should not have any blank boxes unless one of several boxes explains a single care issue. Simply write "N/A" to show that the area was looked at but did not apply to this specific patient care need.

CRITICAL PATHWAYS CHARTING

Critical pathways are commonly constructed using aggregated data of patient responses to expected interventions. Tailoring the needs of an individual patient using a critical pathway might be more difficult when the merging of more than one pathway is required. An example of more than one concurrent pathway is physical therapy's interventions across the same time as occupational therapy and nursing pathways. Recording the time and sequence of interventions, responses, and outcomes using the critical pathways method of recording standardized care is one recording method that is gaining popularity.

According to Sheehan and Sullivan (1997), "When carefully researched, well written, properly followed, and completely documented, critical pathways are a valuable tool for minimizing liability" (p. 123). Some of the issues that remain under scrutiny are the potential liability for the developers of the pathways. Many health care facilities develop their own pathways instead of using copy-righted pathways that might not always meet the protocols practiced by specific physicians.

Another issue in critical pathways is the limitation of information contained within a pathway document. This information might not always contain enough data to demonstrate that the nursing standards of care were accomplished. A major concern is a lack of professional clinical judgment in assessing each individual patient for unique needs (Dykes and Wheeler, 1997).

CONCLUSION

The current approaches in nursing charting are built around the nursing process. The forms are varied and require a broad range of understanding if health care delivery is to be recorded accurately and with minimal repetition. However, sufficient detail is needed to provide information for other members of the health care team to understand the condition of the patient and to have an awareness of nursing or medical interventions that have been or are presently being undertaken. The medical record is a permanent legal record describing the interactions among the health caregivers, health care providers, and patient. Regardless of the recording system used, meticulous and accurate charting is essential to meet the obligations of nursing practice while preventing legal entanglements due to inaccurate or incomplete charting.

CASE STUDY

Mrs. V was taken to General Hospital's emergency department following an automobile accident. She suffered compound fractures of both lower legs and multiple lacerations on her face, arms, chest, and legs. Following several surgical procedures, she was stabilized and progressed from critical care to the general medical/surgical unit.

The hospital used CBE on the nursing units. Every shift, the assigned nurse charted an initial assessment within the first 2 hours of the tour of duty. If nothing had changed with the patient's assessment or condition, then no progress notes were entered into the record.

On the 10th day of hospitalization, Mrs. V complained to her nurse and family members about a general feeling of illness that did not seem to come from the pain and discomfort associated with her injuries. The family asked the nurse what could cause her to feel so badly after 10 days. The nurse told the family that the patient was just now beginning to feel all of the aches and pains of the accident and that the pain medication had been switched to an oral dose that might not provide total relief from the pain. The nurse added that no one wanted Mrs. V to become addicted to pain medicine. The family agreed. Mrs. V continued to experience the general feeling of illness.

On the 12th day, Mrs. V had a temperature of 102°F, an elevation from her 2-day baseline of 99.8°F. Fluids were encouraged by the nursing staff. The nurses listed dehydration from insufficient fluid intake as a nursing diagnosis and initiated a plan of care. No progress notes were charted.

The physician saw the elevated temperature during morning rounds and discussed Mrs. V's general condition with the assigned nurse. A physical assessment was made, and the physician ordered that Mrs. V be taken to a procedure room to open the bilateral lower leg casts to examine the incisions from surgery. On opening the lower left leg cast, a very foul odor was immediately noticeable, followed by purulent greenish drainage. The right leg was healing well.

After several additional surgeries and extensive antibiotic therapy, Mrs. V lost her lower left leg by amputation. The family filed a lawsuit against the hospital, physician, and nurses for failure to properly monitor Mrs. V's condition, resulting in the amputation and permanent disability.

The attorney for the hospital and the nurses argued that it was "uncertain" whether the nurses had or had not observed a subtle change in Mrs. V's condition, but they had failed to record that information due to the charting system. No answer was forthcoming related to the potential actions that might have been taken by the physician if notification of the change in Mrs. V's behavior and complaints had been made. In her deposition, one of the nurses named in the claim said that she would not chart anything that was not a serious change in the patient because she understood CBE to mean that only major events were to be recorded. She continued with statements that CBE was to save time in writing in the chart and that she rarely used the progress notes.

This case was settled out of court just prior to trial. The hospital brought in an educational consultant nurse to initiate an educational program that was mandatory for all nursing personnel. CBE was continued along with a semiannual in-service education review of the use of this charting system.

COMPUTER-BASED PATIENT RECORDS

3

Elizabeth C. Mueth

Chapter Outline

Computer-based patient records (CBRs) are a recognized solution to the increased demand for access and synthesis of patient information. Yet, after 30 years of research and development, and although technology currently is available, the majority of patient records remain paper based. Depending on state laws, patient information must be stored for up to 25 years. Paper records are prone to error or displacement and often become illegible over time. On the average, prior patient records are unavailable in 70% of cases. As a result, in 70% of emergency situations, there is no historic information on patients who cannot answer questions at times when seconds might count (Milholland and Heiler, 1996).

CBRs reside in a computer system specifically designed to support the health care team. CBRs provide access to historic and current health care records including comprehensive clinical financial and research data. In addition to comprehensive patient information, CBR systems provide access to a wide array of support information including clinical alerts, reminders, clinical decision support systems, and links to health care knowledge. Thus, by expanding on the traditional record retrieval and storage system, the CBR meets the information needs of health care providers into the future (Milholland and Heiler, 1996).

TABLE 3.1 Reduction of Administrative Costs

Method	*Benefit(s)*
Reduced redundant data entry	This saves staff time and reduces the potential for errors.
Electronic claims submission	Fewer claims are rejected for clerical errors, and paperwork is reduced.
Improved risk management	Information about errors and adverse events is immediately available. Error-checking algorithms reduce adverse situations. Investigation and evaluation of individual occurrences can identify trends so that preventive actions can be initiated.
Reduced malpractice premiums	Timely retrieval of patient data, decision support, and risk management capabilities provide incentives for insurance carriers to lower premiums.
Reduced storage space	Less physical space is required due to the compact nature of electronic storage.
Faster retrieval time	The person needing the information can access it directly, reducing the need for third-party assistance.
Improved productivity	Because information is correct, comprehensive, and readily available, providers spend more time on patient care and less time on data retrieval.
Financial decision support	Costs associated with health care delivery can be easily analyzed, and data can be retained indefinitely.
Closer connection between provider and patient	The need for repeated patient history is eliminated. Providers and patients can spend more time discussing treatments and responses to treatments. Providers can hold knowledgeable discussions with patients at any time or place. Patients develop a stronger sense of participation in the health care process.

ADVANTAGES OF COMPUTER-BASED RECORDS

CBRs are capable of having many more simultaneous users than are traditional systems. The benefits of CBRs are threefold:

1. Reduced administrative costs (Table 3.1)
2. Enhanced health care research
3. Improved patient care

The most important of the three benefits is improved patient care.

Health care research is enhanced by CBRs, which offer a wealth of information on patient problems, delivery of health care, and outcomes of care.

TABLE 3.2 Increased Access to Patient Data

Method(s)	Benefit
Improved quality of care	Ability to integrate information over time and between settings
Access to knowledge and decision support	External references, full-text literature, research outcomes, and treatment guidelines
Eliminate duplicate diagnostic tests and workups	Current results available at all times, reduced need for repetition
Reduced delays in obtaining test results	Real-time updates, data available as soon as entered
Clinical decision-making capabilities	Instant display and analysis of data accessible by any combination of variables (e.g., body system, date, symptom)
Focus on wellness	Ability to link data on diet, environment, or lifestyle to outcomes and health maintenance issues
Patient care management system	Links to protocols and health care information that allow the computer to suggest additional tests and treatment plans based on similar cases
Integration of data from various health care settings	Improved communication among providers
Direct link to reportable diseases	Reportable diseases flagged in database, can be automatically reported to proper organization when indicated as diagnosis
Organized patient data	Uses a consistent format for terminology and content for ease of analysis and retrieval
Timely data capture	Information collected as events occur

Outcomes can be studied with relation to heredity, environment, or lifestyle. Patterns from institutions or individual practitioners may be analyzed. Longitudinal studies are more easily performed via computers. Research can be used to refine or develop practice guidelines (Table 3.2).

DISADVANTAGES OF COMPUTER-BASED RECORDS

Even the best computer system will have "downtimes" for routine maintenance or system backup (Latz, 1992). Power failures also can affect the availability of a CBR system, as can a limited number of terminals or access points. Methods of recording data during system unavailability must be developed. Data collection forms should follow the same format as does the on-line system. Data should be entered as soon as the system becomes available.

Although not actually considered disadvantages, other issues surrounding CBRs that must be resolved are staff attitudes and training, nursing implications, legal issues (including security), and secondary users of health information.

NURSING IMPLICATIONS OF COMPUTER-BASED RECORDS

The use of CBRs will have a significant impact on the practice of nursing. Much progress has been made in the area of converting charting systems to computer-based records. Nursing has already agreed on a Nursing Minimum Data Set. This, in addition to several nursing vocabularies (i.e., North American Nursing Diagnosis Association, Saba Home Health Care Classification, Omaha System, Nursing Interventions Classification), is recognized by the American Nurses Association for incorporation into a Unified Nursing Language System (UNLS) (Milholland and Heiler, 1996).

In addition to the UNLS, CBRs have a positive impact on nursing productivity and clinical decision making. Productivity is improved through reduced documentation time, faster and simultaneous access to information reducing report time, and more accurate analysis of workload leading to more insightful patient care assignments.

Improved clinical decision making is another result of the CBR. The CBR results in better coordination of care through point-of-care access to patient information and other resources. Nurses are able to spend less time on data entry and more time on analysis and decision making. It should be noted, however, that although the decreased documentation time and increased patient care time do improve the quality of care, they do not allow for increased patient load (Pabst, Scherubel, and Minnick, 1996).

LEGAL IMPLICATIONS OF COMPUTER-BASED RECORDS

Patient records contain personal information. In addition to medical information about the patient and his or her family, the typical record also contains financial data including social security and insurance identification numbers. Summaries of treatment from previous physicians and institutions usually are part of the record. Subjective information, such as physicians' and nurses' notes, descriptions of lifestyle choices, religious preferences, and social history, also may be included. Because all of this sensitive information is critical to the medical record, the issues of confidentiality, privacy, and security are vitally important (Gilham, 1996; Reed, 1994).

Privacy is the right of the patient to govern how information concerning himself or herself is collected, maintained, used, and disseminated. Privacy ensures that information collected for a specific purpose is used only for that purpose, thus remaining confidential. Confidentiality indicates a relationship between the collector of information and the subject of that information. It is the process of maintenance, use, and dissemination of the information. The patient must consent to the method surrounding the use of the information. Security is the method by which confidentiality and privacy are maintained (Reed, 1994).

The advent of the CBR has necessitated new methods for maintaining the privacy, confidentiality, and security of patient information. The basic ethical and legal requirements still apply because, regardless of form, all patient records must be protected. According to Iyer (1991), there are 13 basic charting rules that, if followed, should protect the nurse in case of legal action:

1. Write neatly and legibly.
2. Use proper spelling and grammar.
3. Write with blue or black ink, and use military time.
4. Use authorized abbreviations.
5. Transcribe orders carefully.
6. Document complete information about medications.
7. Chart promptly.
8. Never chart nursing care or observations ahead of time.
9. Clearly identify care given by another health care team member.
10. Do not leave any blank spaces on chart forms.
11. Correctly identify late entries.
12. Correct mistaken entries promptly.
13. Do not sound tentative; say what you mean.

These rules still apply to the CBR. In fact, the CBR solves some of the issues such as legibility, date and time stamps, ink color, and late entries, and sometimes it solves issues such as abbreviations, spelling, blank spaces, and corrections.

In 1973, the U.S. Department of Health, Education, and Welfare developed the Code of Fair Information (Fitzmaurice et al., 1993). It has five main points:

1. Personal data records shall not be secret.
2. Individuals must have access to records about themselves and know why the records are kept.
3. Personal information may be used only for the purpose for which it originally was collected.
4. There must be a mechanism for individuals to correct the personal information in their records.

5. Organizations that collect, maintain, use, or disseminate identifiable personal data are accountable for the reliability and proper use of the data.

CBRs present two unique problems: security of the individual record and security of the personal information contained in the database. Electronic data cannot be locked in a file cabinet in the manner of a paper record. The confidentiality of a CBR is limited by the effectiveness of an electronic security system. The security system is vitally important because CBR systems usually can be accessed from any terminal, often including terminals that are off-site. Such access also may lead to questions concerning the accuracy of the record's contents (Rhodes, 1995).

PASSWORDS

All electronic security systems require some sort of authentication whereby the user must identify himself or herself to access the system. Common methods include magnetic cards, fingerprint recognition, retinal scan, and voice recognition. These methods usually are used on highly sensitive, expensive government systems. Most CBR systems require the use of a secret password (Kibbe and Bard, 1997).

Health Care Financing Administration regulations require that all entries to patient records must be identified as to author, date, and time of entry. Electronic signatures are an acceptable method of identifying entries (Kadzielski and Reynolds, 1993). CBR systems can provide such identification automatically, based on the health care worker's password or sign-on. This makes it vitally important that passwords not be shared with other workers. Such sharing can be active, as in the giving of one's password to another, or passive, as in leaving a terminal unattended after signing on to the CBR system. An unattended terminal can leave patient information displayed where others can see or alter it, thus compromising both confidentiality and accuracy. Entries made during either method of password sharing are not properly identified in the record (Iyer, 1993).

Charting under the password of another means that the owner of the password is credited with all charting entries. This could result in a difficult legal problem. If the patient were to take any type of legal action, then the owner of the password could be held responsible for any actions charted under his or her password. This places the owner of the password in the impossible position of trying to remember everything that happened on the day in question and who might have used the password. The password owner's credibility could be questioned because of his or her allowing the password to be used by others (Grant, 1993).

ERROR CORRECTION

Any entry made and stored to a CBR is considered a permanent part of the record and may not be deleted. It is permissible and advisable to correct any errors before storing the entry. After the entry has been stored, it is important to follow the proper procedure for correcting errors. Just as in a corrected paper record, the CBR should indicate "mistaken entry" followed by the correct information. The corrected entry should be identified by password, date, and time. If information is stored in the wrong record, then the correction should read "wrong chart" followed by the correct identification (Iyer, 1993). The correction never should read "error" because this could be interpreted to mean an error in treatment rather than in charting (Iyer, 1991).

PATIENT IDENTIFICATION

The nature of CBRs requires that each patient have a unique identifier. It has been suggested that a universal identifier would lend itself to tracking health information about an individual throughout the health care system. The least expensive solution to this dilemma would be to use the social security number (SSN). However, there are serious public concerns with using the SSN to identify CBRs. SSNs are already used to identify employment, educational, credit, Internal Revenue Service, motor vehicle, and other personal information. Possible links between health information and any of these other personal records could lead to discrimination by employers, insurance companies, and/or financial institutions based on information obtained from CBRs. SSNs are the most commonly used identification numbers. Public concern must be considered seriously when discussing the benefits of a universal identification number (Fitzmaurice et al., 1993).

CONSENT FORMS

To protect confidentiality and to protect the health care team from unfounded malpractice suits, release forms signed by the patient have become an integral part of traditional medical records. Release forms are required to discuss, copy, mail, fax, or destroy any part of the record. They also are required before many laboratory tests and procedures. The CBR might not allow for hard copy release forms. Computer technology will allow for the ability to input paper documents into the CBR by means such as scanners. It also is possible to input an electronic signature using a slate with a laser pen. Such technology currently is used by some credit card and delivery companies (Tracy et al., 1996).

DISPOSAL OF PRINTOUTS

Just as it is important to avoid leaving a terminal unattended after accessing a CBR, it is imperative that printed patient information be disposed of properly. Once the information is out of the control of the health care worker, there is no control over confidentiality. The procedure for disposal of printouts must be followed meticulously. It is suggested that personally identifiable information be shredded or the identifiers removed or blocked out before disposal. Any private personal information that is forwarded from the CBR system to another location via fax, mail, printout, e-mail, or modem should be marked "confidential," and instructions for proper disposal should be included in the transmission (Tracy et al., 1996).

FIRE WALLS

A fire wall is a computerized access control for a network-accessible computer system. If a CBR system resides on a network that also accesses the Internet or even an in-house network, then it is imperative that fire walls be built. There are many ways in which to accomplish this type of protection. Passwords to the system can be programmed to access only certain areas of the network on a need-to-know basis, thus keeping unauthorized personnel out of the CBR system. The CBR system could reside on a dedicated server where only certain people have access. For systems with modem access, the system could be programmed to "call back" the user at a preprogrammed number. Data transfer over the network or via modem can be limited. Encryption may be used for any type of data transfer so that only those with the encryption "key" can decrypt the information (Kibbe and Bard, 1997). In all instances, access to the CBR system should be monitored for unauthorized access (Waller and Darrah, 1996).

SYSTEM BACKUP

The need for system backup is twofold. First, a backup system is needed for use during system downtime. Even the most reliable of CBR systems will have a certain amount of downtime. Even if there are no technical difficulties, routine maintenance sometimes causes downtime. Maintenance should take place at low use times such as at night or on the weekend. A mechanism to record patient data during downtime needs to be developed. Forms normally are developed for use during these times. Data can be entered when the system becomes available. Second, a complete regular backup of all data is necessary in case of a "crash" in which all or part of the database is lost. Such system backups normally take place daily or more often if the volume of changes to the database is high (Latz, 1992).

There are many uses for medical information that are completely unrelated to any type of medical treatment. Health care workers must safeguard medical records to protect patients from the potentially harmful effects of disclosure to unauthorized parties.

> Individuals have been denied credit, admission to educational institutions, and insurance coverage based on information contained in medical records. Public knowledge of some medical conditions can lead to discrimination in employment, inability to obtain a driver's or marriage license, or missed business opportunities. (Reed, 1994, p. 355)

Administrators of health care facilities have a legitimate need to use information from medical records to assess the quality of health care provided at their institutions. The information also may be used in budget planning, market analysis, and allocation of resources in patient service areas. Third-party payers, such as insurance companies and (increasingly) the federal and state governments, also need access to patient information to assess the viability of reimbursement programs and utilization reviews as well as to protect themselves from fraud. The reliable and easily accessible information in a CBR system is an advantage for these secondary users. Employees of the secondary users must exercise as much caution as do health care workers to ensure the confidentiality and privacy of the records (Reed, 1994).

In the private sector, personal information is not subject to the strict protection it receives in the public sector. As private information becomes more easily collectible and marketable, concern for confidentiality increases. Many private companies now collect, store, and distribute personal information under the guise of service to the insurance industry. Physicians and hospitals are approached to provide information and often do so without notifying their patients (Reed, 1994).

As more institutions convert to CBR systems, it becomes increasingly important to safeguard patient information. Second-party users of information contained in CBRs must provide assurance of anonymity of information, internal and external security, employee manuals detailing security policies, and a "paper trail" that traces transmissions, requests, and access to the system.

GOVERNMENT REGULATIONS

All patients have the right to expect that their medical records will remain confidential and private. This right is protected by constitutional and statutory laws at both the state and federal levels. The right to privacy is not specifically addressed in the U.S. Constitution. However, the U.S. Supreme Court has stated that this right is rooted in the First, Fourth, Fifth, Ninth, and Fourteenth Amendments. The right to privacy, as addressed in the Constitution, includes the right to personal decision making without government interference, prohibition on government disclosure of personal information, and the right to be free from government surveillance of personal affairs (Byars, 1996).

Two federal statutes make limited provision for privacy and confidentiality of medical records: the Privacy Act of 1974 and the Freedom of Information Act of 1966. The acts provide limited protection because they are written to apply to all government records. The Privacy Act regulates the collection of data by federal agencies. Individuals must be notified that data are being collected, the reason for the collection, and whether the disclosure of the data is voluntary or mandatory. Any federal agency that violates the act may be liable for civil actions, criminal actions, or both (Byars, 1996).

The Freedom of Information Act grants public access to all federal records. There are nine exceptions to this access. Medical files are one of these exceptions because public access would be an invasion of personal privacy. To qualify for this protection, three requirements must be met:

1. The information is part of a medical, personnel, or similar file.
2. Public access to the information must constitute an invasion of privacy.
3. Public access must cause an invasion more serious and important than public interest in the information.

The Act also protects medical records from federal drug and alcohol treatment programs. Drug and alcohol records may be disclosed only with written patient consent and then only for specific reasons:

1. Medical emergency
2. Scientific research
3. Audits or program evaluations
4. Court order

The protection from these federal statutes does not extend to state or local government agencies (Byars, 1996).

The Health Insurance Portability and Accountability Act of 1996 (Public Law 104-191) seeks a national health care information database. The Act also requires that standards be created to protect the privacy of individuals. In response, the Department of Health and Human Services secretary, Donna Shalala, proposed on September 11, 1997 that medical information may be released only for purposes of medical treatment or payments. Under these standards, patients would have access to both their individual records and the access logs for those records. Amid concern that these standards do not provide enough privacy protection, Senator Patrick Leahy introduced the Medical Information Privacy and Security Act in the fall of 1997. The bill gives individuals the right to inspect and correct their records and to decide whether and how their information could be released. Civil rights of action are available for misuse of the information (Guard and Langman, 1997).

State protection for medical records is not uniform. However, most states provide some amount of judicial or statutory protection. Constitutional rights to privacy are recognized in Alaska, California, Florida, New York, and South Carolina. Some states have freedom of information acts similar to the federal statute that provide similar protection. California and Tennessee have confidentiality of medical information acts to protect the release of personal medical information without written consent of the patient. Most states protect, to some degree, the privacy of personal medical information. State agencies can face either civil or criminal liability for the unlawful disclosure of personal medical information (Byars, 1996).

CONCLUSION

CBR technology is in a state of rapid development characterized by the constant emergence of new capabilities and applications. The judicial system must provide adequate laws to mediate disputes that recognize these technical advances. As CBRs move toward a national health care database, individual privacy issues are brought to the forefront. Current privacy laws are directed toward the traditional paper record and must be rewritten to include issues that are unique to the technological age.

Security is of vital importance to ensure that records are trustworthy for patient care. CBR systems must be designed and protected to accomplish this goal. Whether the system is electronic or manual, human factors (e.g., errors, negligence, unethical behavior) can result in breaches in confidentiality or inaccuracies of information contained in the record. Ongoing personnel training, regularly updated instruction manuals, well-designed security systems, and strictly enforced security regulations can ensure that a CBR is actually more accurate and secure than a traditional paper record.

COMMON PROBLEMS OF RECORDING IN THE MEDICAL RECORD

4

Sue E. Meiner

Chapter Outline

In Chapters 2 and 3, multiple styles, formats, and systems of recording in the medical record were presented. This chapter looks at the problems commonly encountered in record reviews for litigation purposes. Some of the issues to be presented focus on difficulties in using a documentation system, whereas other issues occur when one facility uses more than one system or mixes systems, formats, or styles on a single patient care unit.

Issues dealing with competence in charting are addressed. Errors, omissions, and alterations of the medical record are discussed in terms of potential liability. Suggestions given in this chapter do not supersede any agency policy or procedures that are in place. However, the information given is basic to proficiency in recording interventions and responses in the medical record.

MULTIFOLD CHART FORMS

Even when a documentation system is effective, the forms that are developed by the facility to meet the needs of the nursing staff, medical staff, and other multidisciplinary health team members can pose problems. The most striking forms that pose difficulties for legal reviewers are the multifold chart pages.

Critical care units in hospitals often develop chart forms that can provide immediate reference to multiple areas of medical, nursing, nutrition, laboratory, and diagnostic test information. These forms are too large and extensive to cover the front and back of a single page (8.5 × 11 inches). Therefore, a substantial number of facilities use the multifold, multiple-page form. This form folds outward from the chart binder up to three folds. As a result of this configuration, material is contained on one continuous form the size of three single pages, front and back.

To save recording time and redundancy of writing, usually only one part has the patient's name, identification number, and date. The concern arises when the form is copied. The foldout pages must be copied separately on most photocopy machines. When this is done, the name, identification number, and date usually are missing from all but one page. This provides discontinuity of information because the pages that do not have identifying data cannot be assumed to belong to a single-face sheet with identifying information.

COMPETENCE ISSUES IN CHARTING

The busy staff nurse does not always have the luxury of recording every event at the time of occurrence and in detail. Good intentions about recording details of care later in a shift have led to many examples of incomplete charting. In the event of a claim against the nursing staff, an incomplete record of patient assessments or nursing interventions can indicate to a jury that the care was not completed. Although this might not be true, an impression that an unfinished entry in a medical record is an indication that care given was sloppy or incomplete may be inferred.

The art of charting develops with practice over time. The method of charting is as important as the content. Defensive charting can be learned with attention to word choice using objective charting.

Subjective and Objective Information

The practice of physical assessment includes obtaining subjective and objective information from the patient. *Subjective* is defined as "perceived only by the affected individual and not by the examiner" (Miller and Keane, 1997, p. 1429). *Objective* is defined as "perceptible by the external senses. . . . a clear, concise declarative statement that directs action toward a specific goal" (p. 1051). Using these definitions as the standards to gauge objective charting

TABLE 4.1 Charting Unfounded Conclusions

At 4 a.m., Nurse Brooks hears a loud noise from a patient's room. When she arrives, Mr. Carl is found sitting upright on the floor and crying. A focus examination is done by the nurse, revealing no apparent injuries and normal vital signs. Mr. Carl is confused as to date and time only, another baseline finding. The on-call resident physician is contacted from the room phone, and she responds quickly. The physician's assessment confirms that no change in baseline data has occurred. The only orders written are for close observation throughout the remainder of the shift and to call the attending physician at 8 a.m. to report the event.

The nursing progress notes are as follows:

6/13/__   0430   Pt. fell trying to get out of bed. Sitting on floor crying, V.S. wnl, no signs of cuts, bruising, or injury, oriented to person and place only, on-call resident notified, responded, orders received. _____G. Brooks, RN

0630   F/u fall: oriented to person and place only, V.S. wnl, no complaints of pain, HA, N/V, incident report to supervisor, verbal report to day shift. _____ G. Brooks, RN

Risk manager's findings:

As a follow-up to the incident report, the risk manager visited Mr. Carl. Mr. Carl was pleasant and alert but did not remember anything from the past night. His roommate, an alert and oriented man, volunteered a statement to the risk manager. He said that Mr. Carl had not fallen but had sat down on the floor to wipe up the spill from the water pitcher that had been knocked off of his bedside stand. The roommate was awakened by the rattle of Mr. Carl's bed just before he saw the pitcher fall to the floor. He witnessed Mr. Carl using the towel that had been on his overbed table to cover the spill. He reported that Mr. Carl then sat on the floor and started to cry.

Jumping to conclusions:

The assumption that a fall had taken place was based on the noise heard and the crying patient sitting on the floor. Without being a witness to a fall, Nurse Brooks could have recorded the objective information beginning with hearing the noise and what she observed on entering the room. The risk manager did not want the mention of an incident report to appear in the nursing notes. Nurse Brooks was assigned to attend an in-service program on charting.

can prevent information based on personal values or feeling from being entered into the record.

Charting nursing care should follow the guidelines that include descriptive, objective data instead of data based on inferences, conclusions, assumptions, and hearsay. Using words that relate what the nurse sees, hears, smells, feels, counts, or measures is objective charting.

During the charting process, the nurse must take time to plan what he or she will enter into the record prior to the actual entry. This can prevent the recording of opinion and the drawing of conclusions that should be avoided in the medical record. Table 4.1 provides an example of an assumption that was written as fact.

TABLE 4.2 Terms to Avoid in Charting

obnoxious	high	disgusting	unintentional
rude	uncooperative	ignorant	error
nasty	discourteous	drunk	wrong
crazy	irrational	miscalculated	accidentally
stoned	bizarre	waste of time teaching	

TABLE 4.3 Items to Avoid in Charting

- Conflicts with other staff members
- Staffing problems, especially too few or a shortage of nursing staff
- Incident reports (when used for quality improvement purposes, some states restrict their use in litigation)
- Incompetence of other staff members or physicians

Charting Negative Opinions

The term *dirty laundry* has a negative meaning when reference is made to recording events in the medical record. Unhappiness on the job should be directed toward employee assistance programs or human relations counselors, not in the written format of the medical record. Disparaging comments about peers, physicians, the patient, or family members are inappropriate in the medical record. Some words can seem unprofessional at best and libelous in certain circumstances. In a circumstance where an untoward event takes place and the medical record is brought before a jury, words that indicate errors by other health professionals or biased feelings toward the patient or family can reflect poorly on the writer. Avoiding words that are derogatory or imply a lack of cooperation is a sound practice for defensive charting. Table 4.2 lists words that are best avoided in charting. Table 4.3 identifies items that should be avoided in charting.

Charting Too Little

Each documentation system has a set of advantages and disadvantages toward general use. Systems that require mainly checkoff flow sheets with only unusual events written in sentence style were established to reduce the time spent on documentation. However, these systems open liability concerns when so little is written that the record cannot reflect occurrences surrounding an actual misadventure or unwanted patient outcome.

ERRORS

Medication errors cover a broad spectrum of mistakes. Errors that can be made include those in transcription of orders, preparation of the dosage or drug, and administration (including the wrong patient) as well as a variety of charting errors. Bernzweig (1996) noted that in hospitals an estimated one of every seven medication orders has an associated error. He added, "In no other area of nursing practice is there a greater need for independent and intelligent judgment" (p. 190).

The transcription of physician orders for medications from a handwritten order sheet to either a computer data transfer system or a paper path to the pharmacy can pose problems. When only one person interprets a handwritten order that frequently is illegible and written in Latin terms or medical abbreviations, errors are more likely. Most systems in the late 1990s have implemented a check and balance for the handwritten orders.

A unit or ward clerk commonly transcribes orders and then passes the work to the registered nurse for review and validation. In some acute care facilities, the pharmacy receives the original order form, with only a copy remaining on the nursing unit. This shifts the transcription to the pharmacy, where an acute scrutiny of the spelling and dosage parameters for a specific patient takes place. However, even this practice can lead to human error when a pharmacy technician transcribes the orders without a pharmacist checking for accuracy.

Errors in the Preparation of Medications

Liability may result from miscalculations of dosages during drug preparation. An example of a potential for errors in preparation is where medication is sent to the nursing unit in a vial of sterile powder that needs to be reconstituted. This usually is done when the time between mixing and delivery of the medication's strength is relatively short. The pharmacy sends the medicine ready for reconstitution into a liquid form. Absolute attention must be focused on the correct reconstituting solution, the correct amount of solution at the end of reconstituting, and the available strength of the final liquid. Then, calculations are needed to determine a dosage after conversions between measuring systems are completed. If this is done correctly, an error still can be made in selecting the appropriate syringe and needle for injection. Another place for errors is in the actual drawing up of the medicine into the syringe. Too little or too much can change the original intent of the physician toward an appropriate dose. At the bedside, the selection of a site to inject the medicine can lead to an error, and the technique for administering the injection can contribute to another error.

TABLE 4.4 Potential Sites for Medication Administration Errors

- Transcription of orders or transmittal of orders to or in pharmacy
- Incorrect mixing, calculating, or preparing of medications
- Incorrect patient or incorrect site/route of administration
- Incorrect charting or marking of fluids, IVPB, or multiuse vials

TABLE 4.5 Medication Timing

O.D. = once daily (or O.D. = right eye)   Q.D.= every day
B.I.D. = twice a day; can be routinely at 9 a.m. and 5 p.m.
Q 12 h = twice a day, every 12 hours
T.I.D. = three times a day; can be routinely at 9 a.m., 1 p.m., and 5 p.m.
Q 8 H = three times a day, every 8 hours
Q.I.D. = four times a day; can be routinely at 9 a.m., 1 p.m., 5 p.m., and 9 p.m.
Q 6 H = four times a day, every 6 hours; can be routinely at 12 midnight, 6 a.m., 12 noon, and 6 p.m.
H.S. = hour of sleep   Bedtime = hour of sleep

Finally, the recording on the medication sheet and in other places, depending on the type of medication, must be completed. Table 4.4 provides a list of these potential points of errors.

If a medication is withheld for any reason, then noting that fact in the chart is recommended. Actions taken to address the omission of the medicine also are needed. If the drug was withheld due to an NPO (nothing by mouth) status, then record the reason and check to see whether an alternate route for administration is acceptable. If it is, then obtain an order from the physician and complete the administration process.

Errors in following the doctor's orders can include the selection of timing for administration of the medication. Frequently, the physician will order a specific medicine to be given before meals and at bedtime. Literally, this is four times a day. But in administration terms, this does not follow a four-times-a-day schedule. This can be confusing for new employees or for physicians new to a facility—or even new to a single unit of nursing care. Table 4.5 provides examples of timing errors that are possible.

The Wrong Patient

To the non-nursing person, administering a medication to the wrong patient might seem absolutely negligent. Although liability rests with the person committing the error, sometimes circumstances need to be reviewed prior to total

---

EXAMPLE 4.1   Misidentification and Potential Medication Error

Mr. Johnson and Mr. Jamieson were patients in a semiprivate room in Good Hope Memorial Hospital. Both men were over 80 years of age and hard of hearing. Mr. Johnson was in the bed nearest the hall door, whereas Mr. Jamieson was in the bed nearest the outside window. The bathroom was in a corner of the room near the hall door. Mr. Johnson left the room to walk his visitor to the elevator when Mr. Jamieson began to walk toward the bathroom. The phone rang, and Mr. Jamieson sat on the bed of Mr. Johnson to answer the call.

Nurse Hart entered the room to administer medications to both gentlemen. Seeing the empty bed near the window, she picked up Mr. Johnson's tablets and approached Mr. Jamieson. She called him Mr. Johnson, and he looked at her and said "yes." When he took the tablets from Nurse Hart, he said "wait a minute" and ended his telephone call. He then told Nurse Hart that he had never taken any of the tablets she had given him before. He questioned her further.

Nurse Hart immediately recognized that something was wrong and asked to see his wristband. When she read the name Mr. Jamieson, she became upset, took the tablets back, excused herself from the room, and went immediately to the charge nurse to discuss the situation.

Result: There was no injury or liability issue, the Quality Improvement Program became involved, an in-service class was held, and no punitive actions toward Nurse Hart were taken.

---

condemnation. Identification bands are supposed to be worn by every patient throughout the hospital stay. Nurses routinely are expected to check the wristband or other form of identification on every patient prior to administering medication. This is to ensure that the correct patient is receiving the correct drug.

As the acuity of patients has escalated, emergency procedures have increased accordingly. It is not unusual to have had to cut off the restricting wrist identification band as a safety precaution during some procedures. To prevent severe constriction of circulation to the hand by the inflexible wrist band, a potential risk for misidentification is created. Example 4.1 provides an anecdotal story of misidentification.

When recording the administration of medication into the patient record, checks need to be made to ensure that the data entry is being made to the correct record. Careful attention to the name on the record is needed prior to recording the medication administration.

Omissions in the Medical Record

Although attention has been focused on medication errors, other errors that can lead to issues of liability include omission of information that could be vital to the medical plan of care. The notification of laboratory reports that are abnormal or of critical values is essential to be recorded in the patient's record. Of importance is the time of the call, the results of the tests, and the person reporting the information. This needs to be followed with the actions taken to transmit this information to the health care provider. Again, the time, information relayed, and person taking the information are essential to record.

If the record is reviewed at a later time to determine when and who received information related to abnormal test findings, then omission can infer that no follow-up was done. If an untoward event happened in which results of laboratory tests were critical but were unreported to the health care provider, then liability will rest on the person responsible for the failure to transmit the data.

Another area of omission to avoid is failure to record preparations for invasive procedures. Preparations can include omitting food and fluids, skin sanitizing, and/or internal preparations such as "bowel preps."

A bowel prep can remove the contents of the intestinal tract through cathartics. If an ordered prep was not done, was incomplete, or was not recorded and an untoward event occurs during an open bowel surgical procedure, then liability may be placed on the person assigned to provide a safe preoperative preparation.

Incomplete Records

Evaluation of the results of treatments or medications is one component of the nursing process. This component will identify the patient's response to medical or nursing interventions. The recording by written statements or the checkoff of a flow sheet indicating that an intervention took place without a follow-up description or acknowledgment of a response may be considered an incomplete record. An incomplete record can infer that no follow-up took place. In the event that the lack of a follow-up led to an untoward event related to a lack of action by the responsible health care provider, liability may be placed on the person failing to pass the information along.

Telephone calls from other members of the health care team, and especially from the health care provider, should be mentioned in the record. The flow sheet format usually has a checkoff for such calls with a space for the time. Other styles may have specific places to list the form of the physician contact and time.

If information is given or received that affects the plan of care, then notation should be made relating those data. If orders are given, then that needs to be indicated. If orders are not received after a contact in which orders were expected, then the notation of not receiving orders should be made.

Orders given over the telephone need to be written immediately. Obtain assistance in carrying out the orders if some must be done without a moment's hesitation, but do not delay writing the orders. In the event of an emergency surrounding the telephone call for orders, transcribing might not be a priority, and the written orders might be omitted from the record. This omission might have occurred so as to provide appropriate nursing care. However, in a court of law, the jurors are skeptical and might not believe or understand the rationale for failure to write physician orders in the record.

ALTERATIONS TO THE MEDICAL RECORD

Alterations can be the result of a simple mishap during handling of a chart or of purposeful destruction or discarding of pages from the medical record. At other times, willful changing of the record takes place to mislead or falsify care that was omitted or was not done correctly.

Common Alterations of Misleading or Falsified Events

Once an error has been identified by a health care professional, action needs to be taken to correct any harm done by the error. Health care professionals are human beings, and errors will occur from time to time. When an error occurs, the patient's safety and well-being are examined immediately. This can be followed by notification of the immediate supervisor to guide the employee through the correct path or an immediate contact with the physician to determine whether any actions are needed as soon as possible to remedy the error. When a cover-up is encountered, the medical records often are quite telling of an error. The orders, actions or interventions, and response to care do not agree with the ultimate outcome. On careful examination, alterations to the medical record often can be identified.

Some of the more common alterations include changing the date and/or time of an event. This could pertain to assessments, medications, or treatments. The next most common finding is the entry that has been written over with darker markings. Adding words or prefixes to words that change the meaning of the notation is another example. Handwriting changes can have several common identifying characteristics such as the following:

1. Handwriting style change in the middle of a single timed entry
2. A single written entry for multiple times during an entire work shift
3. Mark over and mark out of entries made during a period of concern
4. Out-of-order time sequence

Damaged Pages in the Written Chart

Recording in the medical record always requires thought and organization. It frequently is done while sitting at a desk or table. Charting often is accompanied by drinking a beverage. If an accident befalls the event and the beverage is spilled on a page, then entries might be blurred beyond readability. In this event, the original page must be retained (even if dried and placed in a plastic sleeve). The information must be transcribed onto a clean page headed by the notation "copied from page ___." The original page should be retained in the chart in front or behind the recopied sheet. (Procedures may vary by institution. Follow the specific guidelines established in your agency.)

Missing Pages and Chart Thinning

As charts are moved from place to place in a hospital, the likelihood that a page will be lost from the chart is increased. The type of chart binder can make a difference in retaining all of the records. Another risk factor in losing chart pages is with the extensive paper chart that has not been thinned. The process of thinning a chart means to remove data that currently are not relevant to the immediate care of the patient but have been obtained during the current institutionalization. The thinned pages must be maintained on the unit with the active chart. A notation in the front of the active chart must list the content and dates of the material that was thinned.

Charting Others' Work
or Having Someone Chart for You

A nurse charting for a coworker or having a coworker chart for a nurse is a breach of standards of practice. The rule to follow is that a nurse always should chart his or her own actions unless the nurse records an event that describes what was done by another. The patient's medical record is devalued when interventions are interpreted and recorded by someone else as if the care were rendered by that person. The various states' nurse practice acts do not condone delegation of charting nursing care to someone other than the person who rendered that care. Charting hearsay or secondhand information by a nursing professional is questionable at best. Practicing safe and legal nursing implies that the care given is documented by the person giving that care.

CONCLUSION

There are multiple ways in which the medical record can be problematic. Some problems are accidents, some are caused by poor judgment, and others are truly negligent behaviors. The issue of competency of recording in the medical record must be addressed early in the medical employment setting. Orientation programs need to instruct new employees in the charting systems in place and provide a practice opportunity prior to expecting proficiency.

A nonpunitive system of treating medication errors is a must in today's health care environment. The continuous increase in the number of medications that are available, sound alike, and are spelled quite similarly can be overwhelming to health care professionals in a variety of health care settings. Nurses need to remain current on new medications through a variety of continuing education methods. Following a circumscribed approach to medication administration and calculations is a sound practice. When in doubt about a drug or calculation, a safe practice is to check with another nurse or the pharmacist prior to administration.

Recording orders and notes regarding telephone calls to physicians to give a condition report should be charted along with the date and time. Multifold forms need to be examined for adding the name, identification number, and date to all pages. Completing records in a timely manner and correctly marking entries that are mistaken or on the wrong chart usually can prevent accusations of negligence when the medical record is reviewed by an expert witness in the event of a claim of negligence.

CASE STUDY

Mr. W, a 48-year-old diabetic, was admitted to the medical floor of a hospital after being found unconscious at home by his wife. Mr. W's Type I insulin-dependent diabetes mellitus (IDDM) had been very difficult to manage over the past 2 years.

He was placed on an insulin intravenous (IV) piggyback infusion into a main IV line of 1000 cc, $\frac{1}{2}$ normal saline infusing, at 125 cc per hour. Bedside blood glucose (BG) measurements were ordered every 2 hours with a sliding scale insulin order per BG readings.

The evening nurse took a BG reading at 10 p.m. and identified a result that required 15 units of regular insulin. (With insulin being given so frequently on this medical unit, it was the practice not to have anyone else check the type or dosage of insulin prior to administration.) The nurse prepared the insulin appropriately but heard a loud noise and yells coming from a patient's room. She interpreted the sounds as a patient falling. She handed the syringe to another nurse, new to the unit, to administer to Mr. W. The second nurse administered the 15 units of insulin, IV push, as she had done in the emergency room during the care of a diabetic in ketoacidosis. No one charted the insulin. Each nurse thought that the other had charted the medicine. The first nurse accompanied the patient who had fallen to the X-ray department per physician orders. The second nurse continued with her patients. The supervisor took over as a temporary relief for the first nurse. She reviewed the assignment sheet and then the chart of Mr. W. When the BG reading was noted without an insulin administration recorded, she drew 15 units of regular insulin and administered it subcutaneously (as ordered).

Change of shift occurred, and the first nurse returned to the floor to finish charting. She noted that the insulin had been charted by the supervisor and thought that was odd but did not follow up on this unusual event. The second nurse had left and did not have a phone number listed in the unit file, so the matter was ignored.

At midnight, the night shift nurse carried the BG monitor to the bedside but could not arouse Mr. W. An emergency assistant was called. Because Mr. W was breathing and did have a very fast pulse, an emergency call for assistance, or "code blue," was not initiated. When the BG was taken during the emergency care, it was 28 mg/dL.

Mr. W suffered profound brain injury and remained in a vegetative state. The family filed suit against the hospital, specific nurses, and the physician. The physician was released from the suit, but the hospital and nurses were not released.

This case demonstrates multiple medication errors. The extreme overdose of insulin was the direct result of someone else administering a medication that was prepared by another nurse, giving insulin by the wrong route and then failing to chart the drug appropriately, failing to give or receive a status report, and using personnel inappropriately (the supervisor should have taken the patient to the X-ray department)—in general, the breakdown of rules in administration of medication.

ISSUES REQUIRING REPORTING AND RECORDING

5

Sue E. Meiner
With Linda Steele

Chapter Outline

Principles of communication are found in curricula at all levels of education in the United States. Health care providers are presented with multiple opportunities over the years to study and practice the art and skills of communication. Clearly and appropriately communicating with patients and with other members of the health care team concerning patients is essential both to reducing confusion and to managing the risk of malpractice exposure. Communications regarding health care are accomplished in a variety of ways.

This chapter addresses the issues of when and when not to communicate health care data. Information is presented regarding what can be said or written and when the failure to communicate can lead to claims of malpractice, negligence, and breach of standards of care.

A review of the legal obligation of nurses to ensure reasonable and clear physicians' orders and/or to clarify orders that are incomplete or confusing is presented. The issue of reporting medication errors is discussed in this chapter, whereas the recording of errors was presented in Chapter 4.

CONFIDENTIALITY

Written communication in the form of the medical record is a carefully guarded property of health care providers. Black (1991) identified confidential communication as privileged communications between special parties such as a physician or nurse and a patient. It is a statement made under circumstances demonstrating that the speaker intended the statement to be heard by only the person to whom it was addressed. If the communication is made in the presence of a third person not essential to the communication, then it is not privileged.

Medical records include more than just privileged statements between parties. Information obtained by health care team members through observation, assessment, treatment, or conversation also is considered confidential information and is protected by law. The code for professional nurses from the American Nurses Association preserves the integrity of confidentiality concerning all matters that come to the knowledge of a nurse within legal and moral boundaries.

Confidentiality of verbal and written communication within health care is essential to achieve an open dialogue between the patient and the providers of care. The sense of trust between patient and health care provider lies at the heart of the confidentiality concern. The personal and often intimate details of a lifestyle must be freely discussed to achieve an accurate diagnosis and plan of care. Information contained in the medical record is the result of an ethical and legal relationship. Whereas the ethical responsibility for maintaining confidentiality is a long-standing, fundamental health care principle, the obligation to safeguard confidentiality of the medical record is a legal duty (Guido, 1997).

The legal duty to protect confidentiality of medical records is derived from statutory and common law and legally binding administrative regulations. The constitutional right of privacy extends beyond the record and includes verbal instructions of advice and information by health care providers.

The Privacy Act of 1974 protects the rights of patients to have direct access to their own medical records. If release of that information could cause an adverse impact on the physical or mental health of the patient, then disclosure of documents may be denied to the individual requesting them but permitted to a designated physician. Other exceptions within the Privacy Act that affect health care providers include demand for records in the form of a court order signed by a judge, disclosure for a compelling need that can affect the health or safety of others, and reports of communicable diseases and possible abuse (Beckmann, 1996; Bernzweig, 1996).

When Copies of Medical Records Are Requested

Copies of medical records can be requested for a variety of reasons. Requests for copies may be made because of relocation of the patient to another community, change of primary care providers, or a desire to make a legal review for suspected breach of standards of care. Review of the record for purposes of research, data collection, or continuing education reasons, including taking material directly from the record without using the patient's name, is acceptable in most circumstances. This does not constitute a breach of confidentiality so long as the record is used for the intended purposes and the patient's name remains inviolate.

Verbal Disclosure of the Medical Record

If information from the medical record is disclosed without the express consent of the patient, then the institution and the person making the disclosure may be subject to liability in damages. Consent forms for the release of medical record information must be signed in the presence of a witness. The witness will need to sign the same form to validate that the signature was written by the person whose name appears on the form. The signature usually is written in the presence of the witness. Exceptions to this specific process exist when information is obtained with a court order, by subpoena, or by express statutory authority.

PERSONAL INJURY CLAIMS AND RELEASE OF INFORMATION

The plaintiff will be required to sign a release of information so that the record can be reviewed for breach of standards of care in claims of personal injury. In some states, the patient's right to privacy is waived when a lawsuit is filed. This usually is limited to the records pertaining to or surrounding the injuries claimed in the lawsuit.

TELEPHONE TRIAGE

Large numbers of telephone calls to the offices of physicians and other primary care providers made by patients or their caregivers seeking counsel for medical problems are handled on a daily basis. Estimates indicate that from 2% to 28% of primary care given is by telephone (Robinson, Anderson, and Erpenbeck, 1997). Busy office practices are inundated with calls from diverse sources such as frantic parents, nurses caring for home care clients, and others with both emergent and nonemergent situations. Immediate decisions must be made as to the disposition of such calls so that the proper advice may be dispatched in a timely manner. The problem of call-ins has long been a difficult one that can cause harm to a patient and/or place the provider in a compromised legal position.

An accepted definition of *triage* is to sort, to classify, and to choose a path for action based on the first two identifiers. Registered nurses employed in ambulatory care settings, such as physicians' offices, usually are involved in fielding these large volumes of telephone calls from patients. The ability to effectively triage and respond to telephone calls when there is no visual input to assess, and when the reliability of the patient cannot be judged, makes this process very difficult for even the most experienced nurse. Educational background, experience, and inherent personal factors such as intuition, maturity, and people skills influence the nurse's ability to use effective judgment in triage situations over the telephone. Risks are greater because judgments and decisions often are made quickly in a hectic or crisis environment. Nurses, however, are ideal candidates for the decision making required in this process because of their ethical and legal responsibilities in the nurse-patient relationship.

Advanced practice nurses (APNs) are now entering the primary care arena in larger numbers than ever before. They often will answer telephone calls directly, or office personnel who handle the telephones will seek the answers from them. Nurses traditionally are prepared to work in acute care settings, so their basic educational programs and their experience as staff nurses offer little preparation for the in-office scenario in their advanced practice roles as nurse practitioners. To date, nurse practitioner programs have not included this type of content in their curricula to any great extent. Another shortfall occurs in the socialization process of nurses as they are taught to seek the answers and decisions for diagnosis and treatment of patients from physicians (Scott and Packard, 1990).

APNs must be armed with telephone triage skills as a part of their clinical decision-making process so that when judgments must be made in response to office calls, they are well equipped to handle them. In addition to the responsibilities of registered nurses, APNs also will be expected to diagnose and prescribe based on information obtained in telephone interactions. Thus an accurate and comprehensive documentation system will assist APNs in arriving at the best clinical decisions when dealing with telephone calls. Documentation procedures also will help prevent ethical/legal pitfalls that might result from incorrect decisions made when no formal system is in place.

Procedures for handling telephone calls are implemented in a variety of ways depending on office policies. They vary from taking messages to offering advice on many levels. Some advice is given to the caller after an office conversation with the primary care provider. At other times, advice might require the use of complex protocols designed specifically to cover those situations most likely to occur in that particular setting.

One of the difficulties encountered in trying to establish a system of documentation is the variety in types of calls received. Calls can range from requests for prescription renewals, to common complaints of an acute nature (e.g., cold and flu symptoms, sore throat, earache, cough), to those of a more serious but vague nature (e.g., abdominal pain, shortness of breath, chest pain).

TABLE 5.1 Order of Frequency of Telephone Triage Use

1. Abdominal pain
2. Medication prescription renewal
3. Persistent vomiting or diarrhea
4. Bites: insect, animal, human
5. Pediatric rash
6. Menstrual irregularities/vaginal bleeding
7. Pediatric cough
8. Pediatric fever
9. Chest pain
10. Adult rash
11. Eye problems

SOURCE: Adapted from Robinson, Anderson, and Erpenbeck (1997).

Another difficult aspect is that sometimes a seemingly simple request, such as a prescription renewal, can have far-reaching effects. Consider, for example, the case of a 55-year-old woman, with a history of taking estrogen for 8 years, who requested a prescription renewal. The medication could easily be renewed without a chart review if the patient were a longtime patient in the practice. However, an actual chart review revealed that she had not had a mammogram for 3 years. Even though the mammograms had been ordered, each appointment had been canceled by the patient (Emergency Nurses Association, 1991b).

Some health care providers suggest that the simplest solution to a thorny case such as this is not to offer any advice over the telephone whatsoever. Many primary care providers are reluctant to make a diagnosis based on a telephone call because they do not believe that an accurate determination of the patient's status can be made. Others simply refuse to make a diagnosis based on a telephone call alone. Many primary care providers are now charging a fee for telephone consultation, thus cutting the volume of calls and discouraging unnecessary calls. None of these, however, seems to be a realistic or practical solution. The threat of an "abandonment" claim is a drawback to insensitive telephone triage handling. Such approaches also tend to negate the continuity of care in the provider-patient relationship. A system that takes into account both the patient needs and the provider responsibilities is needed.

Managed care organizations (MCOs) and health maintenance organizations have programs set up for telephone advice and health care recommendations. In this context of care, fewer unnecessary trips to an emergency room or to the primary care provider's office is the expectation of the organization's management. For additional information on managed care organizations, see Chapter 20.

Robinson et al. (1997) listed the 11 main reasons why patients use a telephone triage system. Table 5.1 lists the order of frequency of contacts by patients using a telephone triage system.

Terms used to discuss care with a patient over the telephone need to be clear, as simple as possible, and confirmed by asking for repetition by the caller. Failure to give adequate information or warnings, or to explain the risks of noncompliance, must be addressed by the telephone triage nurse. When circumstances of a real or potential emergency are identified by the triage nurse, a referral must be made immediately, with documentation of the circumstances of the call and the follow-up to the call. Lawsuits involving telephone triage health care have focused on the failure to provide patients with adequate warnings regarding the dangers of not complying with the advice given.

A documentation diary or log is a necessity in each setting where telephone triage is practiced. A method should be in place for transferring the information to other staff members for input into the permanent office records and, in the case of a collaborative practice, to the physician overseeing the practitioner's work. This written record will assist in quality assurance by keeping track of calls and allowing users to follow trends in calls and callers. Periodic review of the records will provide an additional mechanism for assessing the accuracy of the advice given. Using a checklist of questions to ask callers prior to advice being given, and using a written procedure protocol to assess the quality of that advice, will provide a means for the maintenance of consistent standards of care delivered by telephone triage. Table 5.2 gives an example of a telephone triage questionnaire.

REPORTING PATIENT'S
CONDITION DURING TRANSFER

Patients frequently are transferred during even brief hospitalizations. The verbal report given to the nursing staff from the transferring unit to the staff of the receiving unit is vital to the well-being of the patient. A clear and concise report contains the patient's name, sex, and age as well as complete vital signs, current diagnosis, treatments, operative procedures, completed diagnostic tests (including any already ordered but to be done by the receiving unit), current physician orders, all medications given within the past shift, any medications due to be given within the next 2 to 4 hours, intravenous (IV) fluids given over the past shift (8 hours), remaining IV fluids that will be infused on the receiving unit, and any IV fluids that will be needed immediately following the current infusion. This report should end with any other information that is relevant to the patient's plan of care.

Failure to provide an accurate and thorough transfer report has been the cause of many malpractice lawsuits. These lawsuits have stemmed from omitting a required treatment or medication, from making an IV fluid error, or from overlooking a physician's order for timely interventions that could lead to a serious compromise in the patient's recovery.

TABLE 5.2 Sample Telephone Triage Record

TELEPHONE TRIAGE RECORD

DATE: ____/____/____; TIME: _____hours

mm / dd / yy   military time

Caller: _____ Current patient: ___Y; ___N

name and relationship to patient

Patient's name: (if not the caller)

_____

Patient's address, zip code, & telephone #:_____

PATIENT INFORMATION:

Reason for calling:_____

_____

Record number or social security number: _____ D.O.B. __/__/____

Current medications: mm / dd / yy

_____

Include all over-the- counter drugs: for pain, fever, stomach, sleep, cough, sinus, bowel, diet, etc.

_____

_____Allergies:_____

Current medical problems: _____

Include: diagnoses from previous visits, any major contributing surgeries

_____

_____

Chart pulled: ____ yes; ____ no

Advice given or protocol/procedure followed: _____

_____

_____

_____

Documentation in chart: ___ yes; ___ no

Warnings given: _____

Referrals: ___ Primary Physician; ___ ED; ___ 911; ___ Hotline; ___ Poison

Control; ___ other Where ?_____

R.N. Signature: _____

check here ___ if continued on reverse side

REPORTING MEDICATION ERRORS

When routine procedures are not followed, medication errors are common-place. Many medication errors go undetected, whereas others are found during routine medical record audits after patients have been discharged or otherwise left the facilities.

Any error in medication delivery must be reported to the physician and the nursing supervisor immediately on discovery. The physician will determine

TABLE 5.3 Nine Common Causes of Medication Errors

1. *Patient identification:* Many names sound and look alike. Ask the patient to state his or her name, and check the patient's identification band prior to administration of any medication.
2. *Similar medication names:* Many names of drugs sound and look alike. Take extra time when preparing drugs whose names look like those of other drugs.
3. *Unfamiliar drug:* Refer to a drug book or call the pharmacist for information.
4. *Illegible writing:* Do not try to interpret an order that is so poorly written that doubt exists about any part of the order.
5. *Confusion over equivalents:* Take time to read the original order and the medication administration record for dosage (e.g., milligrams and milliliters, drams and grams, cubic centimeters and ounces).
6. *Drug labeling:* During medication preparation, read the label three times to make sure you catch any mistakes in look-alike labels.
7. *Multiple tablets/multiple vials as a single dose:* Incorrect transcription of an order can result in an excessively large dose being available. The pharmacy is another check and balance but might also miss an error.
8. *Excessive increase in the dosage:* Rarely are medications given in drastically increased dosages; therapeutic effects are difficult to monitor when radical changes are made. Question the rationale prior to accepting the order as written.
9. *Math errors:* Check and recheck calculations when the dosage ordered requires an unusual calculation. Recheck the placement of the decimal point if the dosage is less than 1.

whether countermeasures are needed to reverse any untoward effects of the medication error. The nursing supervisor will begin a review of the circumstances to prevent a similar error from happening in the future. Table 5.3 lists the nine most common causes of medication errors in health care facilities.

INCIDENT REPORTING

The risk manager will be notified according to the procedure set by the facility. A written report usually is required by the risk management personnel. This report is given various names among different facilities ranging from the original "incident report" to the "event record" or "occurrence report." This report generally is made for quality improvement reasons. The report is not a part of the permanent medical record and should not be used as a disciplinary tool. Any reference in the nurses notes to completing an incident report is discouraged by legal counsel in most facilities (Beckmann, 1996; Guido, 1997). Chapter 4 offered additional information related to the recording of medication errors. Chapter 8 provides an in-depth discussion of the role of risk management and the incident report.

REVIEW OF CIRCUMSTANCES AFTER
A MEDICATION ERROR IS MADE

When the urgency of the medication error is over, a retrospective review of the circumstances that led to the error is needed. Even if a quality improvement team is in place to examine medication errors, the specific care area needs to investigate the matter as well. If one medication error has occurred, then others are possible if the conditions that led to the original error are not fully reviewed. In areas where a high volume of care is being given, particularly involving a high-risk group of patients, careful review should be compulsory.

It is estimated that more than 50% of medication mistakes go unobserved and unreported. Because no exact figures are available, routine chart review can identify frequent errors in the record. Determining whether these errors were simply charting omissions, incorrect charting, or true mistakes in medication administration is important. In most cases, no further investigation is made unless notice of legal action is received.

COMPLYING WITH PHYSICIAN ORDERS

Execution of an incomplete or inaccurate physician's order has led to many errors in treatment or medication administration to patients. Liability for errors perpetrated by physicians frequently is shared by the nursing staff, often arising from prescription of a medication listed in the medical record as having caused the patient an allergic reaction in the past.

Even though the physician bears responsibility for the medical management of patients, the professional nurse is responsible for the interpretation and clarification of the physician's orders. Some orders are written in error by the physician. Other orders are unusual but safe, where the rationale behind the order is given to the nurse when the physician confirms the original order.

Clarifying a physician order is expected when the nurse believes than an error might have been made. If the nurse concludes that an order will do harm to a patient, or if an order is determined to be inappropriate according to nursing standards, then a refusal to follow that order can be made. When this situation occurs, a verbal report should be given to the area supervisor, followed by a written statement that is submitted to the nursing supervisor as soon as possible. The statement must contain the details of the event in careful chronological order. The nursing supervisor will need to resolve the nurse's concern as the questionable order is clarified or changed by the physician (Trandel-Korenchuk and Trandel-Korenchuk, 1997).

Incomplete Orders

When an order is incomplete, the physician must be contacted to complete the order. A complete order requires the name of the drug, the dosage, the route, and the frequency or routine standing times (e.g., B.I.D. [twice a day], Q.I.D. [four times a day], Q 8 h [every 8 hours]) or exact times (e.g., 6:00 a.m. and 6:00 p.m.). The patient's name must be clearly printed on each order sheet. No assumptions should be made regarding the meaning of an incomplete medication order. Instead, incomplete orders should not be followed without completion or correction. An order that contains most of the elements of a proper order but assumes that omitted elements can be determined by the nurse is not complete. When the missing elements are contained in standing or preprinted orders, the written order must state what components of the order are to be taken from standing or preprinted orders.

To demonstrate this point, the following example of an incomplete order is instructive: "Demerol 100 mg IV PRN for pain." If standing orders stated that PRN (as needed) pain medication was to be given no more frequently than every 3 hours and that all Demerol IV medication orders were to be diluted in 500 mg of dextrose 5% in water, then the order would be complete only by combining the elements of the written and standing or established orders. The final change that would make this order complete would be a statement following the original language with "administer according to my standing orders for pain management" and then signed by the physician.

Verbal Orders

Verbal orders often are given by a physician to a nurse during patient visits on a nursing care unit. Although a doctor's orders should be personally written by a physician, events do occur in which the physician must leave before completing orders. In any event, the orders need to be restated to the physician for verification.

Verbal orders should be discouraged except in an emergency situation. The Joint Commission on Accreditation of Healthcare Organizations (1995) recognized that emergency situations might create the need for verbal orders. When verbal orders are obligatory under these circumstances, the signature of the ordering physician generally is required within the next 24 hours. In the event that a verbal order is purposefully not countersigned by the physician, the nurse in charge of the area needs to determine the cause of the refusal. Corrective measures followed by a quality improvement study might be needed. Physicians should be reminded to use verbal orders only in emergency situations.

Verbal orders are not telephone orders and should not be charted as such. Using the initials "V.O." for verbal order and "T.O." for telephone order will differentiate the methods of obtaining orders that are written by the nurse. Both types of orders do require the signature of the ordering physician within a set number of hours according to the policy of the institution. The telephone order most frequently is given after a change in the patient's condition is brought to the attention of the treating physician. This usually is done during hours that the physician is not in the hospital. The chart or file should be flagged to identify that a signature is needed at the next visit.

Transcribing and Checking Orders

Physician orders usually are transcribed by unit secretaries in busy acute care settings. The registered professional nurse is responsible for overseeing that orders are transcribed correctly. This includes oversight reviewing the work of the unit secretary and initialing to show that the orders were reviewed. In this setting, when corrections are needed, the orders can be corrected prior to their initiation.

In some care settings, the nurse has a responsibility to check the previous 24 hours of physicians orders on assigned patients. This is particularly sound in areas where the nursing staff is not consistent. The few minutes spent in this manner might prevent an error in treatment or medication and the resultant harm to the patient.

CONCLUSION

The need for following appropriate guidelines when disclosure of a medical record is requested by the patient, legal counsel, or a court order is a matter that requires serious attention at all times. When legal action is initiated, the rights of confidentiality usually are waived. However, all information furnished in response to a request for legal purposes still should be referred to risk management personnel for dissemination.

The privacy of the medical record has multifaceted implications. In some instances, reporting is mandated over privacy. In others, laws are specifically designed to prevent disclosure of medical record information despite requests to the contrary.

How best to respond during telephone triage of patients by primary care providers has become a major concern in the late 1990s. Managed care contracts have tightly regulated procedures required prior to approval of payment for health care services. Establishing procedures and protocols to guide nonphysician telephone triage is strongly encouraged. Establishing a quality review program to ensure that the needs of patients are met through the telephone triage system is essential to avoid harm to patients and to avert malpractice claims.

Patient condition reports made during a transfer from one area of care to another should be as complete as possible. A clear and concise report includes patient data, current treatments and procedures, and all information related to medications.

Reporting of medication errors is crucial. When errors are made, it sets off a problem-solving procedure. Immediate reporting of any errors must follow a set routine if harm to the patient is to be prevented.

CASE STUDY

Mr. Y was admitted to the hospital for elective surgery. He had experienced increasing pain in his right buttock and leg, with recent onset of numbness and intermittent tingling in his right foot along with poor reflexes in the right leg. He weighed 325 pounds and was 6 feet 4 inches in height. He had a lumbar dissectomy with fusion at the L 4/5 disc (the disk space between lumbar vertebrae Nos. 4 and 5 in the lower back).

The neurosurgeon performed the surgery without complications, and Mr. Y was recovering on the surgical unit. A new second-year resident physician was following the surgeon's patients for post-op care. He wrote an order for Mr. Y to be out of bed and ambulating in his room by 8:00 o'clock. Mr. Y had arrived on the floor at 6:30 p.m. The nurse interpreted the order to mean immediately but did not question such early ambulation. At 8:00 p.m., two nursing assistants were told to ambulate Mr. Y. Although he was very groggy, the assistants moved Mr. Y to the side of the bed, pulled his legs, and pivoted him to a standing position. He could not stand, and he fell forward into both assistants, causing all three to fall to the floor. Mr. Y's incision opened during the fall.

After emergency surgery and an extended rehabilitation period, Mr. Y was able to walk with a significant limp and the aid of a cane. He was unable to return to his usual occupation and claimed damages accordingly.

During deposition, the resident physician stated that he had intended the order to be carried out the next morning by 8:00 a.m., not 8:00 p.m. that night. The surgeon stated that he would have changed that order prior to the next morning because that was not his protocol, and the floor nurses knew he never ambulated a lumbar dissectomy patient on the day of surgery. The surgeon expected the nurses to contact him if any questions arose concerning his patients. The nurse that took the order off the chart stated that she always follows every doctor's orders without fail. She added that it was not her place to question a resident physician.

Nurses are responsible for checking physicians' orders and clarifying any inconsistencies identified. This case involves a lack of communication between a nurse and the resident physician and/or surgeon. As a result of not questioning the "out of ordinary" orders, the patient was grossly injured for life. The use of critical thinking and decision making, based on basic nursing knowledge, includes thinking through the effect of a physician's orders on each patient.

REPORTING HEALTH AND SAFETY ISSUES

6

Sue E. Meiner

Chapter Outline

Communication of medical findings to governmental agencies such as the Centers for Disease Control in Atlanta, Georgia, usually is done in relation to contagious or potentially communicable diseases. This chapter reviews some of the areas of mandatory reporting to public health agencies.

When reports are made to the local or state police, they usually are concerning incidents of criminal behaviors with injuries. These can include cases of suspected physical abuse, reports of potential harm through threats of violence against persons, or suspected substance abuse.

Information related to reporting physical abuse and laws that protect health care providers are covered briefly. Protection against a claim of invasion of privacy when information is given to the police as an act of good faith by nurses or physicians is discussed. Material concerning child abuse or neglect will be addressed in Chapter 13.

REPORTING COMMUNICABLE DISEASES

Communicable disease reporting laws have been compulsory in many states since the earliest days of public health concern. Laws exist for mandatory reporting of infectious disease cases by name, address, sex, age, and other identifying information. Careful attention to requirements of specific governmental agencies is necessary to maintain confidentiality and to satisfy privacy laws. If a report is submitted to the wrong governmental agency, then the event reporter might not be exempt from legal action. The causative organisms of any communicable disease will determine the need for reporting and the mechanism for that report.

A listing of all reportable communicable diseases should be maintained in the immediate environment where treatment may be given. In the case of human immunodeficiency virus (HIV), special legislation has been enacted to safeguard the patient's identity. Rules for reporting cases of acquired immunodeficiency syndrome (AIDS) are present in all 50 states, but their wordings can vary as to the exact protocol for reporting (Guido, 1997).

Communicable diseases need to be fully disclosed to other health care workers having direct contact with the patient. Instituting specific isolation technique and properly placing warning signs are only as effective as the instructions given to all health care workers who might have contact with the patient or the patient's property.

Maintaining records of in-service training on isolation technique for unlicensed assistive personnel generally is handled by the human resources department or by the infection control officer. Each nursing care setting needs to maintain an individual record of personnel having direct contact with any patient on isolation. This unit-based record is a fast track system of identifying personnel in the event of a break in isolation with a nosocomial result.

NOTIFICATION OF FAMILY AND FRIENDS

Health care providers have a duty to inform those having contact with persons afflicted with contagious diseases. These include family members, friends, and health care workers exposed prior to identification of the contagiousness of the patient. However, there is no duty to warn the general public. Although state statutes vary regarding notification requirements, legal action has been taken when a hospital failed to notify a friend who had come in contact with a child diagnosed with meningitis (*Phillips v. Oconee Memorial Hospital*, 1986).

The recording of every dose of vaccine to a child is required under the National Childhood Vaccine Injury Act of 1986. In the event that illness, disability, or death occurs as a result of the administration of vaccine, a report must be filed with the Department of Health and Human Services (DHHS) of the federal government. Information that must be in the patient's permanent medical record includes the date of vaccine administration, the name and lot number of the vaccine manufacturer, the name and address of the health care provider administering the vaccine, and any specific information listed on the information and release form provided with the vaccine. Nurses need to encourage parents or guardians of a vaccinated child to keep the child's records in a safe place for future use. A folder might be presented to the child's parents or guardians for ease in finding these records at a later date.

REPORTING OF NONMEDICAL WOUNDS

Reporting certain types of wounds is required by some states. Gunshot wounds are reportable in nearly every state of the union. Some wounds caused by life-threatening sharp instruments must be reported to the local police department. Self-inflicted wounds are reportable in some states but not in others. The requirements of local law enforcement agencies can be important to know if a nurse should encounter medical situations in which injuries possibly caused by criminal acts are involved.

RESPONSIBILITY FOR REPORTING ABUSE

Every nurse needs to be aware of his or her state's reporting laws and mechanisms when physical or mental abuse is suspected. In 1973, the Child Abuse Prevention and Treatment Act was enacted into law. State requirements to report findings of child, spouse, or elder abuse are present in the majority of states and territories of the United States. Abuse reports supersede confidentiality rights of the patient under the condition known as "compelling state interest." Failure to report suspected cases of child abuse can lead to civil liability and damages.

Reporting and Recording Domestic Violence

A victim of domestic violence can obtain a court restraining order or civil injunction preventing contact by the abuser. Reporting in the medical record the presence of a restraining order is important. Regardless of the manner in which such information is received, quoting the statement reporting the existence of a domestic violence restraining order, followed by the name of the person making the statement, is the most reliable way in which to document such a report. If medical care was being sought for injuries caused by violence, then the police will need to be informed and security placed on alert for potential further violence or danger. Reporting such findings to the next level of authority is strongly recommended.

COMMON LAW DUTY TO WARN

Courts have ruled that health care providers have a duty to warn persons identified as potential targets of harm by a patient. The potential to realize the threat of harm must be credible and real. However, no public disclosure of the threat is to be made. During the past 10 years, the duty to warn against possible harm has been expanded beyond notifying of potential bodily harm; property damage also is covered by warning statutes in some states. In cases where the patients making the threats are not detained in a facility, the duty becomes more of a priority. Throughout the warning process, recording the assessment of potential harm to another person must be explicitly entered into the medical record (Guido, 1997). Careful recording of any patient threats toward others must be taken seriously. Names of those being threatened should be recorded specifically along with quotes of the stated intentions. Each entry should confirm notification to the specific agency and the name and title of the person receiving the verbal report.

If legal counsel is needed prior to making contact with the targeted individual, then action should be taken as soon as possible. Using the chain of command within a nurse's agency is the most acceptable protocol to follow. As a staff nurse, reporting and then recording of events must be made to the nurse next in authority. This might be the shift charge nurse or the section supervisor. The nurse's notes or charting format will need to state clearly the name of the person who received the information regarding the possibility of injury by a patient.

Potential for Self-Harm

Law enforcement agencies recognize another circumstance in which health care providers are obliged to break patient confidentiality and make a report. When an imminent threat of suicide is disclosed by a patient to a health care provider, an immediate verbal report is required. Failure to report can subject the health care provider to civil liability if serious injury occurs to the patient.

Suspected Abuse in the Home Setting

Nurses working in home care or community health settings constantly need to be on the alert for family abuse toward the elderly. Elder abuse most frequently is identified within the home setting. Unfortunately, it is rare that such mistreatment is reported by the abused older person. Fear of retaliation by the family member-abuser may be a major reason. In most states, the nurse's official report of elder abuse is a privileged communication that enjoys protection from legal action by the family. Each nurse must become familiar with abuse reporting mechanisms in his or her state or province.

Careful documentation of the physical assessments of a suspected abused patient should be provided along with notes identifying the person reporting or alluding to the abuse. When the suspected abused elder will not discuss or admit to abuse that is apparent, such hesitancy or denial should be recorded as well. The nurse must use professional judgment in reporting abuse. If a home care nurse is the one observing possible elder abuse, then the task of reporting might fall on the manager or supervisor of the home care agency or community health center.

SUBSTANCE ABUSE

Misuse, abuse, and misappropriation of controlled substances have increased among health care workers in the past decade. Careful observation of rules and policies in the handling of narcotics or other controlled substances must remain a priority on every patient care unit where such drugs are stored and administered.

The Comprehensive Alcohol Abuse and Alcoholism Prevention, Treatment, and Rehabilitation Act of 1970, the Drug Abuse Office and Treatment Act of 1972, and the Privacy Act of 1974 have placed limitations on the access to medical records of drug abuse and alcohol abuse patients. Confidentiality for patients in a facility that specifically treats patients for alcohol and/or drug abuse is mandated unless a patient gives consent to access in writing. The written release must contain the following elements:

1. Identification of the person or program permitted to disclose the information
2. Identification of the person or organization that will receive the information
3. Patient's name
4. Reason for the disclosure
5. Explicit extent of the information that can be disclosed
6. Date of expiration of the release or statement of conditions for revocation
7. Patient's signature with the date

Exceptions to the disclosure requirements exist for purposes of research, audits, evaluation of services, court orders, and medical emergencies. In these instances, the patient does not have to give permission verbally or in writing. Even a court order must meet standards that require a hearing to determine whether the purpose for breach of confidentiality is more important than maintaining privacy.

Coworker Involvement in Substance Abuse

The close relationship that can exist among professional nurses working in sustained employment settings with the same set of coworkers is well-known.

Sometimes, this close relationship becomes one of blind trust. Such loyalty, in the extreme, can conflict with regulations imposed for the greater social good. For example, the policies, procedures, rules, and laws that pertain to controlled substances are in place to prevent the misuse and abuse of drugs.

It is not the intent of this chapter (or book) to describe all mechanisms of misuse and abuse of controlled substances by nurses. It is the purpose, however, to call attention to the serious ramifications when such rules are not followed and improprieties are not reported appropriately to the correct agency. Most state licensing regulatory agencies require reporting, by a hotline telephone service, of any misappropriations, misuse, abuse, or other acts of negligence in relation to drugs.

Policies regarding co-signing wasted doses of controlled substances require one observing such waste to sign along with the nurse who had to waste a part or all of a controlled drug dose. Two nurses are required to be present for the change of shift controlled substance count and to co-sign the appropriate form. In most facilities, only the regular licensed staff on a specific nursing care unit can count and/or record the accuracy of the amount of controlled substances remaining at the end of one shift.

Patterns that ultimately can lead to misappropriation of drugs can form when the standards of practice are not continuously and carefully observed. Passing the narcotic cabinet keys from one nurse to another throughout the shift of duty can result in failure to identify the person withholding a missing dose of drug. Permitting licensed nurses, unknown to the regular nursing staff, to handle controlled substances without some type of a check and balance system is risky. Practices such as always letting the same nurse give injectable narcotics to all the patients on a unit whenever that same nurse is on duty can provide an avenue for misuse.

Whenever failure to follow the controlled substance policies of an institution or agency is known or suspected, a report must be made. Within a facility, the pharmacist and administrator over a given area are responsible for overseeing medication administration. When these individuals are not the reporting targets, the responsible party is identified in the policies and procedures of that health care setting. Agencies that proscribe to the Joint Commission on Accreditation of Healthcare Organizations (JCAHO) guidelines follow a clear chain of command when controlled substances are involved. If JCAHO is not associated with the agency, then the Drug Enforcement Agency will supersede.

Personal Involvement
With Drug Misuse or Abuse

The alarming increase in the number of licensed nursing personnel involved in illegally obtaining, misappropriating, misusing, and abusing narcotics has reached an all-time high. Many states now list the names and actions of licensed nurses found guilty of drug abuse. When a nurse admits to abusing narcotics, self-reporting may save a career and a job. The necessity of seeking assistance for a drug problem is now receiving the attention it justifiably commands as society realizes the threat of drug abuse that comes with the constant interaction nurses experience under highly stressful working conditions. Some reports discuss drug misuse or abuse as an occupational hazard among health care workers. Peers should be available as support persons for any nurse needing to self-report misuse or abuse. Personal and collective encouragement to seek help and submit a self-report of drug abuse can strengthen the profession and (hopefully) begin to reverse the tragic rise in illicit drug use by nurses.

CONCLUSION

Reporting of communicable diseases is compulsory in all states. This mandatory reporting is a matter of public health and safety. To prevent the spread of communicable diseases, childhood vaccinations are required of most persons in most states. Exceptions to the vaccination laws usually involve religious beliefs or allergic conditions. The DHHS maintains a database and will initiate an investigation of a specific vaccine when an untoward reaction occurs.

A little-discussed area of nursing communications concerns the common law duty to warn persons known to have been targeted for harm by a patient. Documentation of threats to another person is critical to proving that release of information was appropriate despite the usual confidentiality rules.

Reporting occurrences of bodily harm or property damage to law enforcement authorities is dictated by the specific policies of each institution. Information regarding to whom reports should be made and mechanisms available for the protection of persons targeted for harm should be covered in orientation and continuing annual in-service education for all nurses.

Case law appropriate to the content of this chapter will not be presented. The nature of reporting the various issues discussed in this chapter rarely relate to written material in a patient's medical record other than by institutional policy.

CASE STUDY

Nurse Lindsay worked in a community-based psychiatric/mental health clinic. She saw patients with chronic emotional problems. As a specialist, she worked with a psychologist 1 day a week. A psychiatrist was head of the clinic and was available for consultations as needed.

Mr. M, a 32-year-old man, had been seeing Nurse Lindsay for more than a year for nightmares, insomnia, and mild depression. He kept his appointments and continued on medication for depression and insomnia. At times, he would become anxious and angry, but he always calmed down at the end of the session.

On one visit, Mr. M told Nurse Lindsay that he learned that his ex-wife was moving in with her boyfriend. He was angry and did not become calm by the end of the session.

The next visit was scheduled, and Mr. M arrived on time. He was calm at the beginning of the session but told Nurse Lindsay that he wished his wife were dead, that he hated her for ruining his life, and that she was the reason he was so messed up. The angry conversation continued throughout the session. Another appointment was made for 1 week later instead of the usual biweekly visit.

On the next visit, Mr. M was more agitated, angry, and accusative of his wife being the reason for his failures in life. He repeated that he wanted her dead. Nurse Lindsay gave him behavioral control homework and told him to call her if he needed to talk before the next week.

Two days after this visit, Mr. M murdered his ex-wife and her boyfriend and then committed suicide. Charges were brought against the clinic, the nurse, the psychologist, and the psychiatrist. The nurse was charged with professional negligence. The clinic accepted responsibility as the respondeat superior and paid an unknown but significant settlement to the families of the ex-wife and her boyfriend.

Many questions were raised pertaining to the nurse's judgment in failing to refer Mr. M to either the psychologist or the psychiatrist due to the change in his behavioral pattern. Other questions were raised in regard to warning the ex-wife of potential danger.

In the circumstances that Nurse Lindsay's practice was limited to chronic but not acutely disturbed patients, she should have referred Mr. M to the psychiatrist for an evaluation following the visit on which his anger included a death wish for his ex-wife. Exceeding practice limits and failing to report a significant change in a patient's condition do not change with practice settings.

PART II

THE BASIS FOR LIABILITY

NURSING NEGLIGENCE ISSUES

7

Alice G. Rini

Chapter Outline

Negligence is the most common theory of liability in nursing, medical, or health care institutional malpractice. It is essentially practice that falls below the accepted standard of care established by law to protect others against unreasonable risk. It is failing to do something that should have been done or doing something that should be done but in an improper manner. Therefore, negligence can be omission or commission. Even though negligence seems as though it could mean anything done in a careless, indifferent, or neglectful manner, it is really something quite specific. Nurses are well advised to be aware of all its elements.

The problems of acting carelessly and establishing fault have a long history in the law. The word *negligence* originally was used to describe a breach of a legal obligation, probably by inadvertence or indifference. It once was asserted that negligence was merely one way of committing another tort (Salmond, cited in Keeton, 1984). Now, however, and for much of the past 100 years, negligence is an independent basis of liability and has its own distinct elements. Interestingly enough, the early use of the theory of negligence was for the liability of those who professed to have certain special knowledge, skills, or competence such as physicians and surgeons as well as other craftsmen (Keeton, 1984). Initially, the law of negligence addressed only affirmative acts and rather than failure to act, according to Keeton (1984)—misfeasance or malfeasance rather than nonfeasance. Eventually, it became clear that certain relationships between parties required an affirmative act to do something and that failure to do it in a proper and timely manner was indeed negligence. Negligence necessarily involves *foreseeable* risk, a possible danger of injury, and conduct unreasonable in proportion to the danger. If there is not a reasonable foreseeability of injury, or if conduct was reasonable in light of what could be anticipated as any problem, there usually would be no liability for negligence. These issues make negligence a controversial issue but a very real one.

An interesting note in the history of negligence is that its rise coincided with the industrial revolution and the many accidents caused by industrial machinery. Those incidents that were intentionally inflicted injuries were clearly differentiated from those that were unintended, and such unintended torts became a major cause of legal action for accidental injury, which remains so to this day (Keeton, 1984). This is particularly true in health care situations today.

TERMS ASSOCIATED WITH NURSING NEGLIGENCE

Corporate Liability

The liability of the health care agency or institution for breach of its direct duty to patients/clients and others includes facility maintenance that avoids unreasonable risk of harm, the provision of an adequate and qualified staff of professionals and ancillary personnel, proper supervision and orientation of all staff members, and the adoption of appropriate institutional policies that enforce all of these requirements. Corporate liability is not invoked for every incident of malpractice within the institution. Rather, it is reserved for situations in which an institution breaches its own duty related to the four requirements just listed or in which the institution knew or should have known about breaches of duty by its employees and did not intervene; the reasonable agency standard applies (Brent, 1997; *Edwards v. Brandywine Hospital*, 1995; *Thompson v. Nason Hospital*, 1991).

Expert Witness

This is a person who, by reason of education and experience, possesses specialized knowledge about a particular subject. Such a person may be called on to assist a jury in understanding certain complicated and technical information generally not within the understanding of the layperson. Persons skilled in a profession often are called as expert witnesses (Black, 1991). Experts are called to identify and explain the appropriate standard of care and how a defendant's conduct breached that standard. Merely testifying that the expert would have behaved differently or that he or she has an alternative preferred approach is not the relevant focus, nor does it establish the generally accepted standard (Diamond, Lawrence, and Madden, 1996).

Immunity

Immunity from suit exempts an individual from liability for his or her actions, or an entity from liability for its actions, because of the existence of certain doctrines or protections. *Charitable immunity* was a doctrine that provided protection from suit for not-for-profit and charitable health care institutions on the following bases: (a) that charitable trust funds should not be used for purposes other than to provide care (with such other purposes meaning paying damages to an injured patient), (b) that beneficiaries of charitable care assume the risk of charitable negligence, and (c) that donations to charities might be discouraged if the charities were held liable and had to pay damages out of the donation dollars they received. The doctrine of charitable immunity is now virtually nonexistent except in a small number of states. *Sovereign immunity* was the doctrine that precluded suits against governmental entities on the basis that suits against the government could distract it from its important work and that to sue the entity that created a cause of action for a wrong on exactly that claim was not logical. Most of these reasons no longer exist; however, some forms of governmental immunity still do exist (Keeton, 1984). Where there still is recognition of these immunities, there is a greater chance that an individual health care provider, such as a nurse, might be personally named in any lawsuit (Brent, 1997). In addition, the *Good Samaritan* statutes provide some immunity for health care providers who assist in emergencies and similar situations.

Negligence

This is conduct that falls below an accepted standard of care. It is the failure to do, or the omission of doing, what is required to be done (Black, 1991).

Personal Liability

This is a situation in which a person is specifically liable for actions because of an obligation to do something now or in the future. The person is risking personal loss if there is failure to perform the action. The responsibility is able to be enforced by law, that is, a lawsuit or legal action against the person who failed to perform appropriately or to perform at all (Black, 1991).

Res Ipsa Loquitur

This is a Latin term meaning "the thing speaks for itself." It is an inference that a defendant is negligent because there is proof that the instrumentality causing injury or the situation in which the injury occurred was in the defendant's exclusive control and proof that the accident or injury that occurred was one that ordinarily would not have occurred in the absence of negligence (Black, 1991).

Respondeat Superior

This is a Latin term meaning "let the master answer." In certain cases, a supervisor may be responsible for the wrongful acts of a subordinate, or a principal may be responsible for those of an agent. Inappropriate or inadequate care on the part of a subordinate toward someone to whom the supervisor owes a duty of care will raise the theory of respondeat superior. It applies only when the subordinate is acting within his scope of employment or authority (Black, 1991).

Tort

This is a civil wrong perpetrated by one party against another, other than a breach of contract, for which the law will provide a remedy for the injured party to seek redress or money or other damages. It is a violation of some duty owing to a plaintiff, with such duty arising from the operation of law and not by mere agreement of the parties (Black, 1991).

Vicarious Liability

This is indirect legal responsibility such as an employer's liability for the acts of an employee (Black, 1991). Employers who have neither acted negligently nor intended the action may be liable for their employees' negligence (Diamond et al., 1996).

NURSING NEGLIGENCE

The Elements of Negligence

Negligence as a cause of action has four elements. Each must be present and proven to establish a case for negligence. An inadvertent or indifferent act, although likely reprehensible in the eyes of most nurses, in and of itself is not legal negligence. The four elements are as follows.

Duty. This arises when the relationship between individuals imposes on one a legal obligation for the benefit of the other. It also deals with particular conduct in terms of a legal standard of care that describes what is required to meet the obligation. Duty, therefore, is the requirement to conform to a standard of reasonable conduct in light of the apparent risk. The general idea is that a court will find a duty where reasonable persons would recognize it and agree that such a duty exists (Keeton, 1984).

Breach of duty. This is the failure to adhere to the standard of care, the failure to provide the appropriate care in a timely manner, or the omission of care that should have been provided. Whether a breach of duty occurred or not is based on published standards such as those promulgated by licensing agencies and professional organizations, on published institutional policies and procedures, on expert testimony from qualified experts who can attest to what should have been done in the situation, or by the application of common sense, not necessarily from experts (Trandel-Korenchuk and Trandel-Korenchuk, 1997). A breach of duty can be established from the nursing record that should reflect an assessment of the patient and the care provided in response to that assessment and/or in response to appropriate medical orders. The record should further describe the patient's/client's outcome as a result of the care and any other subsequent action on the part of the health care team. In the absence of any such information in the record, a breach of duty could be inferred because there is no evidence that any assessment or care was provided. There is some belief that if something was not written as accomplished, then it can be assumed that it was not done. Documentation in a patient record also should conform to agency policy concerning such matters.

Injury. Some injury or loss to the plaintiff/patient must be shown. Such injury may be physical, mental/emotional, or financial. There must be evidence of the injury or loss at the time the suit is brought. Physical injury and financial loss subsequent to negligence usually are fairly clear; however, mental/emotional injury is not always so clear. Some courts will permit suits based only on mental/emotional injury; others will allow such suits only if there also was a physical injury or a financial loss (Trandel-Korenchuk and Trandel-Korenchuk,

1997). The most important concept to understand here, however, is that without some type of injury, negligence cannot be proved.

Causation or proximate cause. The plaintiff/patient must show that the breach of duty was the cause of the injury of which the plaintiff complains. Proof is adequate if the plaintiff demonstrates that *but for the action of the defendant,* there would be no injury. Sometimes, proximate cause is difficult to prove because injuries might not be close in time to an improper act, and often a plaintiff's/patient's bad outcome that occurs subsequent to an experience with a health care provider or agency is not related to a breach of duty by the provider.

Proving Negligence

The four elements must be proven by a *preponderance of the evidence,* that is, more than 50%. A preponderance of the evidence means that the greater weight of the evidence favors one side or the other. Where the evidence for one side has a clear superiority over the other, it has nothing to do with the number of witnesses or the pieces of evidence. The evidence with greater weight will show clarity of knowledge, extensive information, a convincing manner, and confidence in the testimony (Keeton, 1984). If evidence includes the medical/nursing record, then the same evaluation of this written evidence is done. Therefore, where documentation is clear, adequately described, convincing, and done with confidence in the accuracy of the data, it is more likely than not to carry the weight of evidence. The conduct of a recent deposition of a physician is illustrative. In this case, a patient had complained of lower back pain and some numbness and tingling in his legs. Over a period of months, he visited an orthopedic physician. During each visit, the patient saw a nurse, who did an initial examination, and then the physician. A review of the patient's medical record revealed that for 14 visits, there were only three notations about the level of pain, whether or not there was numbness or tingling, and how the patient was perceiving his problems. The nurse's notations included vital signs and little else; the physician's notations mostly indicated "no change" or comments that the patient was not yet a candidate for surgery with no supporting data. The deposition was very difficult for the physician and the nurse, who could not justify their lack of adequate documentation of the patient's condition. Because the patient was suing for failure to properly diagnose and treat, and because he subsequently saw another physician and had back surgery, much of his case centered on the lack of adequate assessment and treatment. The nurse and (particularly) the physician were unable to defend their care because there was no documentation of their observations, which would have been essential given that the physician continued to assert that she did not consider the patient as needing surgery. It is clear that in this case, the principles of clarity of knowledge, extensive information, a convincing manner, and confidence in the testimony were absent.

Prevention of Negligence

The four elements of negligence should be clearly understood by nurses who provide care to patients/clients. Prevention of negligence is the best way in which to avoid legal difficulties, and in addition to actual completion of appropriate care for clients, proper documentation of that care, observations pursuant to providing the care, and the responses to care all should be entered in a timely way in the medical/nursing record. Proving negligence generally means that a plaintiff must show that the defendant nurse *physically* failed to do something with the client that should have been done or that the defendant nurse did something incorrectly. The failure of proper documentation might not seem like a negligent act. The preceding illustration concerning the patient with back pain makes clear that although the lack of documentation in this instance might not have been a negligent act in itself, it was so inadequate that it could not support the subsequent action (or inaction in this case) of the health care provider. Therefore, the physician's inaction eventually was found to be negligent enough to cause her to have to pay damages to the patient. If the documentation of the patient's ongoing condition had been clear and convincing, then it is likely that this physician would have avoided liability because her decisions could be demonstrated to be based on observed physical phenomena. It might have been that when the patient finally saw the second physician, his condition had deteriorated to the point where he needed surgery, but it was too late to argue that point at the time of the lawsuit.

Failure to Properly Document Care

Documentation in the client record is primarily a communication tool that ensures that all members of the health care team are aware of the client's progress and that appropriate continuity of care can be maintained. The importance of this communication cannot be overstated. For example, suppose that a nurse administers medications to a patient, records these in a timely manner, and later observes that the patient has had an untoward reaction to the drugs. The nurse discusses the problem with the patient but does not record either the character of the untoward reaction or the discussion with the patient. The nurse has the *duty* to administer the medicine correctly and to communicate to others that it was done as well as any patient outcomes that are material to the continuation of care. Failure to record appropriately and thereby communicate is a *breach of duty,* and a reasonably prudent nurse would know this. It also is reasonably foreseeable that failure to document the patient's problems with the drug could result in another nurse, perhaps on a different shift, again administering the medication without the knowledge of potential problems. If a second dose of the medicine is given with a subsequent untoward reaction, then the *injury* is the second untoward reaction of the patient. The *proximate cause* of the untoward reaction was the failure of the first nurse administering the medicine to record the information about the patient's reaction to the drug, which would alert the rest of the staff to the potential problem, after which it is probable that the offending drug would be discontinued and an alternate prescribed. (It should be understood that notification of the physician also is incumbent on the nurse who observes such an untoward reaction to a medication.) It is not a direct cause because the second nurse actually gave the second dose. However, causation need not be direct. If the "but for" analysis is used, then it can be seen that but for the failure of the nurse to record the patient's reaction to the medicine, the patient would not have received the second dose and, therefore, would not have experienced the untoward symptoms. The actions of the second nurse are important as well. However, the "reasonably prudent" standard is considered. Does the reasonably prudent nurse administer an ordered medication if there is no information that would preclude such an act? The answer probably is *yes*. This might be a question for experts. How far is the nurse in such a situation reasonably expected to go to determine whether any ordered treatment or medicine has caused a problem? If there is no notation of problems in the record, then it is reasonable to expect the medication to continue to be administered by other nurses.

The Substantial Factor Theory

There is another interesting and evolving legal theory of causation in negligence—the substantial factor test. Proximate cause is based on the premise that there is one cause of an injury. Substantial factor permits multiple causes of a particular injury. This theory permits a finding of liability if a defendant's conduct is a material element in causing the injury to the plaintiff (Keeton, 1984). It could be argued that in the preceding situation, either nurse, both nurses, or neither nurse could be proved liable for the injury (untoward reaction to the second administration of an ordered medicine).

The first nurse gave a dose of the medication with no knowledge of the problems the patient would have, discussed the ensuing problem with him, and then failed to document all this information except that the patient received the drug. If the injury complained of was the second untoward reaction, then the first nurse might not be responsible because he or she did not administer it. To find the first nurse liable, a connection would have to be made between the second untoward reaction and the first nurse. The failure to communicate by documenting and reporting the patient's problem with the drug is presented as that connection and, therefore, can be considered a material factor in causing the injury. The second nurse gave the second dose after noting that the first nurse had given the first dose and had noted its administration and nothing else. But it was that second dose that actually caused the injury. Because the first nurse had, in fact, discussed the problem with the patient, was there any responsibility on the part of the second nurse to discuss the medicine with the patient prior to its administration? If this is asserted, then it would be a requirement of *any* medicine ever given to a patient *at the time of administration.* Most nurses probably would say that this is unreasonable. Actually, any case against the second nurse is very weak but not nonexistent.

If the substantial factor test is used in this case, then the connection between the first nurse and the injury can be maintained. Again, if the first nurse had documented the untoward reaction, then it is highly likely that no subsequent doses would have been given. The failure to communicate by documentation and reporting is a substantial factor in the continued administration of a drug that elicited an untoward reaction in the patient. It might be argued that the patient had some responsibility to inform any caretaker that he had some problem with a medicine in the past, notification of which would have alerted the second nurse and likely forestalled the problem of the second dose. But in the American health care system, patients usually are not held responsible in this manner.

Problems in Causation

There are several questions in determining cause. Many courts have adopted the substantial factor theory as a result of the manner in which they address negligence. At one time, most state courts applied the law so that in the case of a plaintiff (the injured party) who did not contribute to his or her problem, the court or jury would find the defendant (the one who did the act or omission that "caused" the injury) wholly liable for the plaintiff's injury. Negligence in health care situations generally does not attribute any contribution to the patient except in noncompliance cases, and sometimes not even with these latter situations. Some states, however, have adopted a *comparative negligence* standard that permits a court or jury to apportion fault among plaintiffs and defendants based on how much each contributed to the outcome of the acts or omissions.

The questions then become the following: How much or what part did a defendent's conduct play in bringing about the result or injury? Was the second untoward reaction reasonably foreseeable as a risk of the conduct by the first nurse when he or she failed to document the problem when it happened? Put another way, could the first nurse have predicted that additional doses of the same medication would be given by others if they did not know that the patient had a problem with it? Should the first nurse be relieved of liability because the second nurse actually gave the dose that caused the injury? Could the first nurse shift liability to another person who had a greater responsibility to protect the patient?

In this case, the first nurse failed to document the untoward reaction, the second nurse gave the medication without checking with the patient about his possible problems with any medications, and the patient did not inform the second nurse (or anyone else) about his earlier problem with the medication. A logical analysis would point to the first nurse, who by an appropriate action—documentation—would have prevented all the following problems. There is support for this analysis. A California court stated, "Foreseeability is not to be measured by what is more probable than not but includes whatever is likely enough in the setting of modern life that a reasonably thoughtful person would take account of it in guiding practical conduct" (*Bigbee v. Pacific Telephone and Telegraph Co.,* 1983, p. 947).

With regard to the actions of the second nurse, it could be questioned whether the second administration was a superseding or an intervening cause. Unless a force or action is highly improbable or extraordinarily *unforeseeable,* it will not be considered superseding and will not preclude liability. One court commented, "If the intervening act is extraordinary under the circumstances, not foreseeable in the normal course of events or independent of or far removed from the defendant's conduct, it may well be a superseding act which breaks the causal nexus" (*Derdiarian v. Felix Contracting Corp.,* 1980, pp. 666, 670). The continued administration of the medication is not highly improbable. In fact, it is highly probable in the absence of information that would alert one to withhold it.

The theory of vicarious liability may shift the burden of protection of the patient from the nurse(s) to the institution or agency in which the injury took place. Actually, the institution cannot insulate itself from liability for the acts of its employees acting within their scope of employment. Even an institution that has policies in writing, in-service education for safety procedures, and other quality management practices ultimately is responsible for the negligent acts or omissions of employees including professionals who are independently licensed such as nurses. The doctrine of respondeat superior holds the employer responsible for such acts and omissions. The law has evolved over the years to treat the employer as having final responsibility for employees acting on its behalf even when an employee violates clear policies. It is seen as the price of conducting the business of the enterprise. Even though the employer can be held responsible for the patient's second untoward reaction to the administered drug in the preceding situation, it does not mean that the entire burden of liability is shifted. Nurses still are responsible for their own acts.

DOCUMENTATION AND NEGLIGENCE

The Purpose of Documentation

Documentation of patient/client care is a tool to provide for the continuum of care that is necessary for quality care and to prevent negligence. Without documentation, there is no way to communicate with other members of the health care team, no way to provide for a permanent record of the care of the patient, and no way to prove that certain aspects of care were provided and what the outcome of that care was. Risk management and quality improvement departments also use the information in the patient record to evaluate care and the need for improvements and changes and to identify areas of potential risk to the institution (Brent, 1997). Every agency and health care institution has policies about documentation because it is so important to the proper functioning of the agency. Some institutions require thorough and specific documentation of care and the activities and outcomes related to that care. Others recommend a minimum of documentation, perhaps with the idea that less writing will give an examiner of the record less with which to work, resulting in less trouble. Documentation also is regulated by governmental agencies, accrediting organizations, and the standards of professional societies. Case or common law also addresses documentation in health care (Brent, 1997).

The Uses of the Patient Record

In addition to the health care provider institution itself, the patient record is used by third-party payers to determine if and when care for which they will pay providers was provided. Others who may use the record include researchers, governmental and private statistical management agencies, accrediting agencies, grantor organizations, and other health care administrative agencies (Brent, 1997).

The use of the patient record that many nurses and other health care providers fear is use in a legal proceeding, perhaps against the nurse or the institution. It is then, of course, that one of the strictest tests of adequate and accurate documentation occurs. Nurses should understand that the patient record is the first piece of evidence that is obtained and reviewed extensively by a plaintiff's attorney (Brent, 1997). In fact, in depositions of nurses, the first questions by a plaintiff's attorney generally ask about the institution's policy about documentation, how well the nurse understands it, and how it is implemented. If the nurse cannot answer these questions promptly and confidently, it is a sign that the institution might not have provided adequate information to its staff, that it might not have regularly evaluated the staff compliance with the documentation policy, and that what will be found in the actual recordings by nurses and other providers will not be supportive of assertions of proper care.

After ascertaining the substance of the documentation policy and the nurse's understanding and implementation of it in the deposition, a plaintiff's attorney will then ask about the actual recordings in the chart. A thorough record of the patient's experience with the health care institution that is accurate and clear will be the nurse's strongest defense against allegations of negligence. Conversely, where the record is incomplete with essential information missing, it is likely that the plaintiff/patient will be able to support his or her claim of negligence. The case of the patient with back pain, described earlier, is illustrative here.

The Extent of Documentation Required

There is some controversy over what and how much documentation is enough and thorough as well as how it actually reflects the aspects of care and other data necessary for the various users of the patient record. An interesting example of this issue is whether or not so-called negative charting is necessary or appropriate. Negative charting is the recording of information about a patient that reflects outcomes that might have been expected but did not happen. There is the case of a postsurgical patient who had been assessed after returning to his room from the postanesthesia unit and was found to have no bleeding from the surgical wound. How many further notations should be made to indicate the lack of blood on the dressing? If a later review reveals no further comments about bleeding, then does the lack of data about bleeding mean that there was none and that the first assessment information had not changed? Or, could it mean that no one ever checked the patient after the first assessment? This latter interpretation is the most likely one if the patient later has a problem with excessive bleeding and experiences a medical injury that might return him to the operating room or to some more grievous outcome. A simple flow chart that permits a quick check mark reflecting not only the observation but also the patient's condition is one of the ways in which to address this problem. There are few legitimate excuses that a court would recognize for failure to adequately document essential information, even if it reveals the lack of a problem.

Another example is the patient who had been receiving oxygen for an extensive period of time. Yet, for several shifts, no information about the route, instrumentality, or flow rate was in the record. There was some question about the adequacy of care related to the oxygen treatment, yet no one could say confidently what actual care was provided. There also was no support for any recollection a nurse or other provider might have because the patient record was silent on this aspect of care. This is damaging to the nurse and to the health care institution, and it is strong ammunition for a plaintiff who brings a negligence suit against them.

PRIVACY AND CONFIDENTIALITY

Privacy

Privacy is a constitutionally protected privilege. It originally was identified as arising from the Fourteenth Amendment to the U.S. Constitution and other language therein that is said to protect personal liberty and freedom from intrusion into one's private affairs. The concept of privacy deals with four major issues: using a person's name or likeness (picture) without consent, unreasonably intruding into a person's private affairs or places, publicly disclosing private facts that ordinarily would be considered private, and putting a person in a false light (Rini, 1998).

Documentation in a patient's medical record can violate privacy if it interferes with any of these liberties. Although invasion of privacy is not negligence, it is discussed here because nurses might inadvertently violate privacy because of a lack of knowledge of the concept of privacy. Violation of privacy is actually a quasi-intentional tort, meaning that although it might not be done intentionally or maliciously, the actual act that constitutes violation is intended, even though an actual injury might not be intended. But it is not done accidently or by mistake.

Violations can occur in the following ways. Showing a patient's/client's picture to other potential clients to induce them to choose services from the agency that generated the pictures is using a name or likeness if done without consent of the person photographed. Unreasonable intrusion can occur if patient care is observed by others who have not been given permission to observe. Releasing patient information to others who have no need or right to know this information is inappropriate disclosure. Writing opinions or making disparaging remarks about a patient/client that become public or influence the impressions of other health care providers about the patient could be considered a privacy violation of putting the patient in a false light. Such comments not only are inappropriate in normal documentation in any case but also can expose the nurse and the institution to legal difficulties (Brent, 1997).

Confidentiality

The concept of confidentiality relates to the expectation of a patient/client that his or her medical and other information will be kept in confidence. This concept supports the notion that a patient will be more likely to share all pertinent information about himself or herself if the patient knows that it will not be released to anyone not involved in his or her care (Brent, 1997). This promotes positive provider-patient relationships and should increase the quality of care.

Anything that one reads in the patient's record is subject to the requirement of confidentiality. Anyone who is authorized by the agency that creates or maintains the record is subject to the requirement of confidentiality, and the number of persons so authorized is increasing with the expansion of the entities involved in the health care system.

STATUTE OF LIMITATIONS

This is the statute or law prescribing limitations to the right of action on certain described causes of action. It bars suits unless they are brought within a specified period of time after the right of action accrued (Black, 1991). The time limit varies based on the type of suit (Black, 1991). In medical or nursing negligence cases, the statute of limitations generally is for 1 or perhaps 2 years. The purpose of such a limit on the time to bring a legal action is to prevent long periods of time to pass before acting because evidence becomes stale and witnesses become unavailable. In negligence or medical/nursing negligence, the statute of limitations runs from the time the injury occurred or from the time the patient should have known of the injury using reasonable diligence.

There are exceptions to the statute of limitations. Minors may be permitted a longer time to take legal action, and if there has been fraud or attempted concealment by a defendant, then the statute may be extended. If such fraud or concealment can be proved, then courts generally will not permit the defendant to use the statute of limitations to avoid the suit or will stop the running of the time to the point of the plaintiff's discovery of the injury.

A good example of the application of the statute of limitations is the case of a woman who had a baby delivered by caesarian section. Apparently at the time of the surgery, two sponges were left in her abdomen. She complained of lower abdominal discomfort for 2½ years, visiting several physicians to attempt a diagnosis. No one was able to identify the cause of her pain, often attributing it to the scarring of surgery. The caesarian section was the only surgery she ever had. The woman again became pregnant and had an uneventful pregnancy except for somewhat increased abdominal discomfort as the pregnancy progressed. At the time of delivery, she had another caesarian section, at which time the two sponges were found walled off within her abdomen. The "abscess" was removed. The hospital and first surgeon settled with the patient on money damages that covered her physician visits for 2 years plus some additional amount for her pain and suffering.

It is interesting to note that when the original chart was obtained for examination of evidence of the operative record and the sponge count, it was listed by the nurses as correct. No charges of fraud were made.

CONCLUSION

Documentation is an important tool in the prevention of charges of negligence. Following the policies of the institution or agency in which one practices is of great importance, and agencies are well advised to adhere to the documentation rules of accrediting bodies and professional societies. These rules are considered evidence of a standard of documentation. Proper documentation is intimately related to continuity and quality of care.

CASE STUDY

A young man broke his leg while playing soccer and was brought to the hospital, where he was seen in the emergency room and then sent to surgery so that a cast could be applied to the leg. Over the next several days, the patient complained of pain under the cast. At one point, the physician cut the cast in several places to relieve pressure. The patient's toes, which protruded from the cast, became swollen and dark and then eventually became cold and insensitive. The nurses documented their observation of the leg, toes, and other data a few times each day. Noted were the presence of blood and other fluid on the cast as well as a bad odor. Eventually, the patient was transferred to another hospital, where he was found to have extensive tissue damage to the leg and infection. He eventually had part of the leg amputated. Testimony at trial established that the damage was caused by the pressure of the cast. The plaintiff also claimed that the nurses and the first hospital were negligent in documenting the problems with the cast and with the patient's leg as well in failing to report the lack of any treatment to forestall the continued damage. The court found that the physician, nurses, and hospital were liable for the patient's injury. The court addressed the failure to more regularly document the progress of the patient, the failure to report the problems (particularly that no action was taken to ameliorate the pain, pressure, odor, and other problems with the patient's leg), and the failure to adhere to an appropriate standard of care related to these issues.

In this case, the issues of reporting and recording were in question. At point is the requirement to do more than write an assessment about a patient problem. The nurse must have an action to resolve or to attempt to resolve a patient problem that is not acted on, in the nurse's judgment. Recording in the patient's record telephone calls to obtain action and the results of the calls must be done with objectivity. Reporting a problem that is not acted on, by a physician or other health team member, to the next person in authority is expected behavior of a professional nurse. However, the transfer of information to the next level of supervision needs to be observed for action. This is where the "chain of command" comes into play. Although this can be problematic, pursuing action beyond the next level must be done with diplomacy while following the agency's policy, procedures, and guidelines of behavior.

RISK MANAGEMENT AND CLAIMS PREVENTION

8

Alice G. Rini

Chapter Outline

Risk management, although a somewhat newer function in health care, has been in place in many industries since the early 1900s. Its purpose is to reduce unplanned financial losses to the organization. The role was a response to a changing legal and work environment in which issues such as workers' compensation, product liability, premises liability, and other general liability were expanding. The idea of quality assessment and improvement is inherent in risk management because it is logical to conclude that high-quality care and maintenance of standards will result in fewer claims for error resulting in loss to the agency.

THE ROLE OF RISK MANAGEMENT

Responsibilities of Risk Managers

To understand the role of risk management, it is important to know the definition of unplanned loss. Such loss encompasses those incidents and occurrences that are known to occasionally happen but cannot be predicted with any accuracy. Predictable losses are those that can be determined by financial planning or the measurement of other standards. Failure to serve an adequate number of patients in a specialized clinic resulting in inadequate revenues and financial loss because the clinic was too specialized is such a predictable problem that is not within the purview of the risk manager. However, the risk management department is responsible for a lawsuit against a health care institution because of a patient fall. Although it is generally known that patients do fall, it cannot be predicted with any accuracy when falls will happen or how many times such incidents will occur.

Although there are health care risk managers in small medical practices as well as large medical centers, much of the more well-known work of risk management occurs in health care institutions. The expanded liability of health care institutions is the result of judicial enforcement of the industry's own best vision of quality practices and accountability (Rosenblatt, Law, and Rosenbaum, 1997). This expanded liability also can be interpreted as a trend toward protecting patients from injury in institutions engaged in risk-creating activity. Rosenblatt et al. (1997) indicated that there is evidence that institutional efforts to provide such protection by using quality and risk management programs have not always been highly successful, reflecting weaknesses in the system. These authors further showed that as health care institutions were better developing their quality and risk management programs, they experienced a reduction in reimbursement for care from governmental and private insurance sources, particularly managed care organizations. This no doubt limited the resources that could be dedicated to quality and risk management efforts because such efforts did not always show an improvement in net profits. Rosenblatt et al. submitted that there are efforts being made that will include managed care organizations in the chain of responsibility for quality of care provided pursuant to their guidelines and financial incentives.

Managing Risk Through Insurance

Risk is managed through some form of insurance. Health care institutions may pay premiums to commercial insurers for such coverage, or they may self-insure. Self-insurance is a system in which an institution formally sets aside funds in an account used for paying claims up to a certain dollar amount as primary coverage. For additional security, they also carry a product called *excess insurance* that covers the cost of claims in excess of the primary coverage. This is similar to carrying a high deductible and, therefore, often is more cost-effective for institutions. The excess insurance policy has a lower premium because it does not cover first dollar lost, so the insurance company is not liable for many small claims that may inure to an institution and pays on behalf of the health care institution only when a claim or lawsuit exceeds the institution's self-insured level (Kraus, 1986).

Using the various forms of risk management, an institution may choose to have a variety of insuring opportunities. With self-insurance, the institution retains the risk and pays claims either from operating funds or from a special set-aside fund for that purpose. An important feature of self-insurance is that the risk manager retains managerial control of the funds and the process by which they will be paid for a claim. On receipt of a claim or the notice that a suit might be forthcoming, the risk manager must make a determination of what the claim might cost the institution whether it is settled prior to trial or it were to go to trial. That dollar amount is then set aside in case the institution must pay certain amounts to the claimant or for a damage award at trial. With a commercial insurer, the institution transfers liability for payment of claims to another entity but loses some control about how and for how much claims are paid (Kraus, 1986).

Whatever the type of insurance, documentation of the insurance provisions, limitations, and exclusions is essential. Insurance companies will not pay claims that fall within the policy exclusions. Not only must risk managers be aware of such policy limitations, but they must inform all personnel such as nurses and other professional health care providers who may be involved in or become aware of events that might give rise to institutional liability. Such personnel should have information in writing, as in employee handbooks or policy manuals, about the type of insurance an institution carries, what measures must be taken if an event that could possibly generate liability occurs, prohibitions, and what type of documentation should be generated about the event and what to do with such documentation.

RISK MANAGEMENT PROCESSES

Identification of Risk Exposure

Identification of risk exposure is an ongoing process. There are so many functions and activities within health care institutions that a risk manager, even one with a staff of specialists, cannot know and be able to analyze all the risks in every area of the institution. Many risk managers use experts within and outside of the institution to assist in the identification and control of risk areas to protect their institutions from financial loss.

Risk exposure may come from a variety of loci within and without the institution. Nurses working in any health care setting might not be aware of the plethora of sources of liability. Table 8.1 shows common risk exposure in health care facilities.

To monitor all the areas from which liability and loss can originate, the risk manager could document, through the use of flow charts, weaknesses in the system processes that could precipitate liability. The documentation of activities and adverse occurrences to determine when and under what circumstances problems occur, and whether or not injury results, can help to predict the most likely time for such problems. This will allow adjustments to be made in staffing, monitoring, activities, or some other factor to prevent injury and loss.

TABLE 8.1 Common Risk Exposure in Health Care Facilities

- Professional malpractice by physicians, nurses, and other practitioners
- Injuries to patients, visitors, and others during their time in the institution or on the grounds
- Corporate liability for the improper actions of employees
- Theft of drugs, equipment, and other institutional property
- Theft or embezzlement of money
- Workers' compensation awards for employee injuries and employment-related disease
- Chemical and other hazardous materials and waste
- Defamation actions
- Antitrust actions
- Actions against directors and officers in their official capacities
- Fraud and abuse actions by governmental and other insurers
- Securities violations associated with institutional funding
- Labor issues associated with hiring, promotion, or termination
- Loss of key employee or intellectual property

SOURCE: Adapted from Kraus (1986).

It is vitally important that these data generated on flow charts, and the analysis thereof, be treated as highly confidential information that belongs only to the institution. Nurses and others who have participated in the generation of data and/or their analysis are cautioned not to discuss the findings from such documentation with anyone outside or inside the institution if that individual has no need to know such information. Nurses should be part of the risk management process, but if there is concern that they will not maintain the confidentiality of the data, then risk managers will be very reluctant to include them in data collection, documentation, or the generation of solutions.

Nurses want to be involved in clinical and practice decision making, so they must act responsibly in such situations. Political attitudes that often are espoused in colleges and universities do not always support the advocacy or advancement of the corporation or institution for which one works. Preservation of financial assets is somehow thought to be less than altruistic. It should, however, be recognized that the financial health of the provider institution is intimately involved with one's continued employment and its ability to care for clients/patients. Therefore, efforts made to improve the quality of care, thereby avoiding the risk of loss from any source, should be supported.

Risk Prevention

Much of the activity of the risk management department is to prevent situations that expose the institution to risk of loss through efforts such as educating personnel, promoting safety in all areas of the organization, and enlisting the help and cooperation of key and other employees in risk prevention activities. Promotion of safety is a diverse function, ranging from the management of hazardous waste to the maintenance of floors in a dry condition when visitors coming in from the rain make the floor wet and slippery. Nurses and other employees have the responsibility of reporting unsafe conditions immediately. This probably would be a verbal report, but it might be prudent to follow up with a written note because documentation of the observation of and subsequent amelioration of the hazard is a helpful item to have if any question of injury or liability were to arise.

Risk Management and Quality Improvement

No discussion of risk management can be complete without some discussion of quality improvement. Although the primary focus of risk management is loss prevention, it should be evident to anyone in the health care industry that losses cannot be adequately prevented unless the quality of client care and of all institutional processes is high. In an ideal situation, risk management and quality improvement should complement each other.

Because risk management came late to the health care industry, and quality improvement was already in place, the two functions remain separate in many institutions. It is likely that this results in duplication of documentation for many situations, particularly those related to client/patient care. Quality improvement personnel often do not see the importance of the non-patient-related issues with which risk management must grapple. Yet, any activity in a health care institution can affect client care. It is time for nurses and other patient care personnel to recognize this. Another factor that affects the relationship between risk management and quality improvement is the timing of their activities. Risk managers are concerned with preventing risk and, therefore, with preventing loss; they also are concerned with the aftermath of adverse occurrences. If an injury or accident were to occur, then the risk manager must act to minimize the financial loss to the institution by mitigating damages or forestalling a claim. Quality improvement personnel are primarily concerned with increasing the number of positive outcomes of client care. They are most concerned with identifying best practices and ensuring that everyone uses them. When there is an adverse occurrence, quality improvement personnel certainly use the information to instruct and improve but then generally pass the problem to the risk manager.

Patient Records Management

The patient record is a tool used in both risk management and quality improvement functions. Failure of adequate and accurate documentation in such records is one of the biggest problems with which these departments have to deal. The role of the patient record is important in the monitoring and measurement of cost, quality, productivity, resource use, and adverse occurrences. Much of the care provided never is documented. This is a problem for measuring service use and productivity. Patients' relationships and communication with physicians, nurses, and other caregivers rarely are documented, possibly because such activities and the recording thereof are not valued or are perceived as less important than recording physical signs and the care provided for them. Yet, there is evidence that there is some relationship between effective documentation and high-quality care (Lyons and Payne, 1974).

Another important reason for having adequate and accurate documentation of all elements of care is to ensure appropriate reimbursement by insurers to the health care institution. It is possible to experience financial loss because care provided was not documented. Furthermore, if a request for reimbursement is not supported by the written record, then an institution could be accused of fraud. For governmental payers, an accusation of fraud by a health care institution has significant financial implications. There is, no doubt, too much fraud in health care reimbursement claims, and this has resulted in a concerted effort to detect the perpetrators. Where documentation is not clear, or where it raises questions of whether or not care was actually provided, there is a great chance that reimbursement will be denied and that an accusation will be made. If there is actually a finding of fraud, then health care providers may be excluded from government insurance programs, such as Medicare and Medicaid, and fines may be levied.

Whereas all record keeping and documentation should be done with the utmost care, if there is an adverse event, then the accuracy and thoroughness of the patient record is of greater importance. It always is a good practice to document with the assumption that the record will be seen by a court; if there is any suspicion that such may be the case, then it is wise to review the record for accuracy, signatures, and other required information. Risk managers usually prefer to separate the chart from the other medical records to preserve it in its original condition. The chart also should not be widely available. It is not uncommon for a plaintiff's attorney to request copies of the patient record at the time he or she is retained. The attorney will later compare his or her copies with the original chart to see whether changes have been made. Changes most likely will be interpreted by a court and/or a jury as fraud and deceit, and often the substance of the case will then be disregarded (Kraus, 1986).

COMMUNICATION, REPORTING, AND DOCUMENTATION

The success of any risk management program is dependent on a timely and accurate flow of information; the generation of appropriate reports; and the documentation of loss prevention activities, adverse occurrences, and investiga-

tion and management actions related to those occurrences. All such documentation also must be maintained in a manner to avoid its release to parties who
should not have access to it.

The risk manager should cultivate as many sources of information as
possible. Nurses, for their part, should view risk management as an important
part of their role and assume the responsibility for being communicators. Early
and effective intervention with patients or others who have experienced problems in the institution or related to any contact with it is essential. Both formal
and informal paths of communication are necessary to manage that early
intervention. Nurses can play a big part in supporting the efforts of the risk
manager.

Clearly, the first responsibility is to provide all formal documents, completed
accurately and objectively, in a timely manner. However, even before the formal
documents can be generated, certain issues should be informally reported
immediately. Such occurrences include falls or other injuries experienced by
patients or visitors, complaints or threats of lawsuits, contacts from attorneys,
media inquiries, unusual incidents, and problems with mechanical equipment
that interfered with patient care. To be sure, there are additional routes through
which these issues should be reported such as supervisors and nursing managers.
Nurses with information should use the appropriate reporting channel consistent
with institutional policy. Nurses should, however, assure themselves that information actually gets to the risk manager in case someone in the reporting chain
misconstrues the gravity of the occurrence. Actions in response to problem
occurrences always should be coordinated with the risk manager so that all
personnel in the institution act in concert with a common goal.

The formal reports that document the information on which the risk
manager bases action remain the foundation of the risk management process.
Words used to describe these reports have been modified from the term *incident*
to give them a neutral tone and not engender anxiety in personnel or give patients
and others a negative impression. Terms such as *occurrence* and *variance* may be
used to describe the events to be reported. In truth, it is not only adverse events
that should be formally reported, but anything that is out of the ordinary course
of events in a particular area of the institution. If nurses are in doubt, or if a
policy manual does not give adequate guidance, then the risk manager should
be consulted about whether a formal report should be generated. Although many
of these reports are generated in contemplation of future litigation, some provide
quality management/improvement information and are necessary to the ongoing
growth of the institution.

One of the important issues that is raised in terms of occurrences that
potentially generate institutional liability is how to deal with the distribution of
such reports. Courts have said that documents prepared for defending a claim
and in contemplation of litigation are not discoverable; that is, they may not be
used as evidence in a trial. The more the institutional process treats the report
of the occurrence as an internal communication to the institutional counsel, the

greater the chance that its nondisclosure will be respected. Therefore, there should be a specific and strict policy about how the report is handled, who should see it, and who receives a copy of it. Many institutions limit distribution to the risk manager or legal counsel and the administrator responsible for the department or area in which the event occurred. Nurses should be aware of the policy and adhere to it without deviation. It is well established that such reports never are attached to the patient record. This does not mean that documentation of any occurrence or experience of a patient is not done. Recording of appropriate observations, assessments, and actions related to the occurrence in the patient record is required. As with any other documentation, recording of an adverse occurrence should be completed objectively and unemotionally.

In the interest of objective reporting, as well as generating data that is able to be computerized, many risk management departments use a coded report form. Such a coded report also provides for improved legibility over a handwritten narrative form, more comprehensive information because the writer responds to questions or information areas rather than trying to determine what to report, more objectivity because data are reported by checking appropriate fields within categories that describe the event and the parties involved, and reduced chance of missing essential information. Coded forms usually provide some space for narrative reporting of information that might not be clear or in sufficient detail in the coded areas. Nurses who deal with occurrence or variance reports should follow institutional policy regarding their completion.

CAUSES OF MALPRACTICE ACTIONS

The law of negligence and tort litigation have affected the quality of care and the deterrence of activities and behavior that could result in injury (Rosenblatt et al., 1997). There is, however, some disagreement about the extent of the impact on health care malpractice, particularly that of physicians. Many physicians believe that malpractice judgments are the result of skillful plaintiff's attorneys and a legal system that favors the emotionally attractive injured patient. In fact, of 100,000 discharges from hospitals, approximately 4,000 patients experience adverse events, one quarter of which were the result of medical malpractice. The 1,000 malpractice-related injuries result in 125 legal actions against health care providers. Approximately 60 patients eventually get some compensation for their injuries, generally prior to trial; only 5 win at trial (Rosenblatt et al., 1997). Documentation of improper practice and of malpractice awards should be able to be used for a quality feedback system, a process that also would contribute to loss reduction.

A study of medical error (Bosk, 1981) identified three major categories of malpractice. One was technical error, in which the practitioner lacked the requisite skill needed to perform the procedures done. The second was judgmental error, in which an incorrect or inappropriate course of treatment was recommended. There was some thought that judgmental errors might have been reasonable decisions at the time they were made or with the information available, but nevertheless, patient injury resulted. The third category was called *normative* by Bosk (1981). This type of malpractice is the failure to perform with the appropriate professional role expectations. Care that was rushed, inattentive, or careless fell into this category. Bosk found that none of these errors was communicated to the patient and that the only reporting, if any, occurred among the physicians themselves. A similar categorization of malpractice was identified by Kravitz, Rolph, and McGuigan (1991). They found three broad areas: patient management problems including miscommunication, technical performance problems, and medical and nursing staff coordination problems.

With regard to nursing malpractice, high-risk areas included improper or inadequate assessment and history taking, technical errors in procedures, failure to follow legitimate physicians' orders, nonreporting of deviations from accepted practice, inadequate supervision of patients resulting in injury, and failure to seek medical attention for patients in a timely manner (Northrup and Kelly, 1987).

CONCLUSION

It might seem that to manage a risk-free environment, there is an overwhelming amount of documentation needed. Although there is a rather extensive role for timely, accurate, and complete record keeping in the area of risk management, it should be approached with logic. Where possible, checklists and flow charts should be used for ease and time conservation. Professional employees are more likely to complete forms that are clear and easy to use. All staff members who are involved in the activities of the organization that might expose it to risk should understand the importance of documentation and plan for it in their time management. It would be unfortunate to be enlightened about the importance of documentation while defending actions that were not reduced to writing contemporaneously with the event.

CASE STUDY

In *Darling v. Charleston Community Memorial Hospital* (1965), an 18-year-old broke his leg while playing football and was brought to the emergency room of Charleston Hospital on November 5. He was treated by Dr. Alexander, who was on emergency call. Traction and a plaster cast were applied. Shortly thereafter, Mr. Darling began to complain of great pain in his toes, which also became swollen and dark in color. They later became cold and insensitive. The next day, Dr. Alexander notched the cast around the toes, and the day after that, he cut the cast up three inches from the foot. Then, on November 8,

Dr. Alexander split the sides of the cast with a saw, cutting the patient's leg on both sides. The odor from the leg now extracted from the cast was very bad. Mr. Darling remained in Charleston Hospital until November 19 and then was transferred to Barnes Hospital in St. Louis, Missouri, where he had several surgical procedures in an attempt to save his leg, all of which were unsuccessful. Finally, Mr. Darling's leg was amputated 8 inches below the knee.

In a subsequent lawsuit, Dr. Alexander paid $40,000 in a settlement. The hospital paid $110,000 pursuant to a jury award. The court described the verdict as follows: The hospital was negligent in allowing Dr. Alexander to do orthopedic work as needed in this case without adequate supervision and by not requiring him to keep his operative skills up to date. The nurses failed in their duty to watch the protruding toes constantly for color, temperature, and sensitivity; to check for circulation; and to report the patient's problems as they unfolded to the appropriate supervisor. The hospital failed in its duty to have an adequate number of appropriately skilled nurses capable of recognizing the progressive deterioration of the patient's leg and of reporting same to appropriate medical personnel in a timely manner.

Darling is the landmark opinion in establishing the idea of corporate liability for hiring, supervising, evaluating, and ensuring that persons practicing within the institution are sufficiently skilled to carry out their duties.

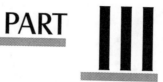

DOCUMENTATION
IN PRACTICE SETTINGS

STAFFING AND DELEGATION OF PATIENT CARE

9

Robyn Levy
Sue E. Meiner

Chapter Outline

The health care environment of today is multifaceted and continues to grow more complex than was imagined even a few years ago. The quality of care delivered is challenged today by serious business considerations such as downsizing and financial cutbacks facing hospitals daily. The necessity of adequate staffing in the face of a continually changing patient census has made the provision for safe patient care a challenge for the administrator and the caregiver alike. Maintaining the nursing standards of care for all patients is the ultimate goal of nurses, health care supervisors, and administrators (Murphy, 1994).

PERSONAL LIABILITY FOR NEGLIGENCE

Accountability for one's actions is at the heart of potential personal liability. Individual or personal liability is based on the concept of fault. For a nurse to be held liable for an act, the nurse must have failed to carry out an act or have done something incorrectly (Trandel-Korenchuk and Trandel-Korenchuk, 1997). Nurses face potential liability every day they care for patients. They are expected to have a level of knowledge and skills that a prudent nurse of the same background would exhibit in similar circumstances (Yocke and Donner, 1992).

Staff nurses must know their environment and work setting if patient care is to be rendered within the expected standards of care. When patient assignments are made at the beginning of a tour of duty, familiarity with the patient population and the unit environment should be addressed. Ketter (1994) reported a set of guidelines to be followed prior to accepting an assignment, as follows:

1. Clarification
2. Assessment
3. Option identification

Clarification means an understanding of the expectations of the assignment. To clarify an assignment, the nurse should learn the situation regarding patient acuity, number of patients assigned, and type of support personnel available.

Assessment means doing a thorough review of one's personal skill levels, knowledge, and experiences and then comparing that information with the environment in which the nurse will care for the patients. Based on this assessment, the nurse must contemplate any risks that might be posed for the patients.

Once the circumstances have been clarified and assessed, it is incumbent on the nurse to know what options are available. If the assignment is accepted, then the nurse will be held responsible for the nursing care delivered (Ketter, 1994; Pruett, 1993).

A registered nurse (RN) has an obligation to refuse an assignment when a patient(s) is (are) placed at risk. Notification of refusal to accept an assignment is mandatory to provide administration an opportunity to look for options to cover the refused assignment. Being able to state correctly the facts concerning the assignment in question to the nurse or supervisor responsible for assignments and staffing decisions, in a timely manner, is crucial. The proper steps must be followed to avoid the accusation of patient abandonment. By formalizing notification to those persons in charge of staffing, a shared responsibility will be established, and accountability will be spread between the nurse and the supervisor as well as the institution.

ASSIGNMENT DESPITE OBJECTION

The American Nurses Association (ANA), as well as many state nurses associations, has taken a position in favor of a nurse's right to accept or reject an assignment. The Missouri Nurses Association has developed a formalized Assignment Despite Objection form (Table 9.1) that can be obtained and used by nurses when the following situations exist:

1. When nurses are expected to assume responsibility that exceeds their experience and/or educational preparation
2. When the volume of care is more than the nurse can administer safely
3. When an assignment is beyond the legal scope of nursing practice

The ANA's (1985) Code for Nurses supports the right of a nurse to refuse an assignment based on the nurse's ethical beliefs. The Joint Commission on Accreditation of Healthcare Organizations (JCAHO, 1996) standards require a hospital to have a policy identifying patient care situations that might conflict with the cultural values and ethical/religious beliefs of the staff member and ways in which requests can be initiated, reviewed, and acted on by the institution. Nurses must take it upon themselves to be aware of their institutions' policies and to follow them. To avoid conflicts, a statement in advance concerning the nurse's position against performing certain procedures or care would be beneficial. A supervisor is better equipped to avoid conflicting assignments when a nurse's beliefs are known in advance. In the case of an emergency, a nurse must administer care regardless of any conflicts that might exist (Davino, 1996).

THE FLOAT/PULL ISSUES OF STAFFING

Adequate patient care staffing is the responsibility of the health care corporation. The legal doctrine regulating this responsibility is the Corporate Negligence Doctrine. This doctrine is not discussed here, but the issues are presented.

The potential for holding an institution liable for negligence in the event of inadequate staffing exists. For liability to arise, a patient must have sustained an injury that was linked to the facility's inability to provide adequate skilled or unskilled staff for safe patient care (Murphy, 1994).

Three different issues concerning staffing were identified by Guido (1997). The first is the ability to provide adequate staffing in light of high patient acuity amid a reduction of financial resources available to the facility. Institutions are obligated to uphold a reasonable standard of care despite staffing problems. Health care institutions are required by the JCAHO and other accrediting bodies to have adequate numbers of qualified staff. Courts have leaned more toward the professional judgment as to what constitutes staffing sufficient to provide safe, prudent patient care rather than following rigid patient-to-nurse staffing ratios. A resultant injury based on "short staffing" and not the action of any one staff member would have to be proved for the nurse manager to be held liable (Guido, 1997).

PURPOSE

The purpose of this form is to notify hospital supervision that you have been given an assignment which you believe is potentially unsafe for the patients or staff. This form will document the situation. Your SNA may use it to address the problem. INSTRUCTIONS: PLEASE PRINT, ONE OR MORE RN's MAY COMPLETE THIS FORM. Send/copy to Missouri Nurses Association, P.O. Box 105228, Jefferson City, MO 65110, one copy to your supervisor, one copy to facility and keep one copy.

Section I: *Before assuming the assignment and completing this form, you must give your supervisor (not the charge nurse) notice of your objection to the assignment. Please put the complete name and title of the person making the assignment and receiving objection. Please complete the response section with the supervisor's response as well as the date/time of the response. If you do not receive a response from your supervisor, submit a copy of this completed form to the next level(s) of administration. Complete the sections "Other persons notified" below if you notified any other persons (head nurse/clinical manager of the unit).*

I/WE _____

Registered Nurse(s) employed at _____ on _____
    Facility   Date   Shift

hereby protest my/our assignment as: ____ Primary Nurse ____ Charge Nurse ____ RN pulled to unit ____ Other

made to me/us by _____ at _____ despite my objection.
                 Superior's Name / Title   Date / Time

Response: _____

Other persons notified: _____ _____ _____
                              Name   Date / Time   Response

_____
        Name

_____
Date / Time

_____
Response

Section II: *Please check all appropriate statements:* I am objecting this assignment on the grounds that:

____ Staff not trained or experienced in area assigned.
____ Staff not given adequate orientation to the unit.
____ Inadequate staff for acuity (short staffed).
____ The unit was staffed with excessive registry.
____ The unit was staffed with unqualified personnel
____ or inappropriate ____ of personnel
____ New patients were transferred or admitted to the unit without adequate staff.

____ The assignment posted a serious threat to health and safety of staff.
____ The assignment posed a potential threat to the health and safety of patients
____ Staff involuntarily forced to work beyond scheduled hours.
____ Other (please explain) _____

106

Section III: Complete to the best of your knowledge the patient census at the time of your objection. From your assessment, indicate for each acuity level, the number of patients on the unit fit into that category. If there are acuity factors not listed, please specify what they are.

Census and Acuity

Patient Census: Start _____ End _____ Unit Capacity _____ Admissions _____ Discharges _____

Acuity Levels: High _____ Average _____ Low _____

Factors influencing acuity. Check those that apply:
___ On respirators; ___ Complete care; ___ On isolation precautions; ___ Restrained; ___ Immediately postop (less than 4 hrs.)
___ Require vital signs/nursing assessment more frequently than routine ___ Receiving blood product transfusions
___ Receiving IV drug/TPN/chemotherapy infusions
Other (specify) _____ Other(specify) _____

Section IV: Complete to the best of your knowledge. Patient Care Staffing Count

	RN	LPN	AIDE	OTHER	CLERK/SECRETARY	PREVIOUS NUMBER OF STAFF OR EQUIVALENT CENSUS/ACUITY
start of shift						
end of shift						

Section V: Complete this section if you think the situation cannot be explained adequately in Sections II and III, or if you think additional information is relevant. Brief statement of problem: _____

As a patient advocate, in accordance with the Nurse Practice Act, this is to confirm that I notified you that, in my professional judgement, this assignment is unsafe and places the patients or staff at risk. I indicate my acceptance of the assignment under protest. It is not my intention to refuse to accept the assignment and thus raise questions of meeting my obligations to the patient or of my refusal to obey an order, which were given; however, I hereby give notice to my employer of the above facts and indicate that for the reasons listed, full responsibility for the consequences of this assignment must rest with the employer. Copies of this form may be provided to any and all appropriate State and Federal agencies.

_____ _____
Nurse's Signature Print Name

TABLE 9.1 Assignment Despite Objection
SOURCE: Missouri Nurses Association (1996). Reprinted with permission.

107

The second issue concerns the floating of staff from one area or unit to a different unit or service setting. The staff nurse has a responsibility to the institution to float to another unit if that unit is short-staffed or if the originating unit is overstaffed. The risk of liability does increase when nurses are unfamiliar with a nursing division to which they float or have less expertise in the care of the population on that particular nursing unit (Guido, 1997).

One critical factor to consider when looking at the issue of floating is the orientation of the pulled staff to the unit. Many nurses surveyed in the Service International Employee Union's 1992 National Nurse Survey (Lepler, 1993) felt that the orientation they received when pulled was not adequate and placed them in unsafe situations. A survey of 319 RNs and licensed practical nurses (LPNs) in Wisconsin voiced this same concern (Nicholls, Duplaga, and Meyer, 1996), with the most common complaint about floating being inadequate orientation. The nurses had doubts that their assessments were adequate and free from omissions or mistakes. Those surveyed felt strongly that they were a burden to the floor staff familiar with the unit and that their presence on the unit was seen by the floor staff as unwanted. It is essential to train and orient float nurses to environments that could become alternate assignments. A receptive environment in which the assistance of float staff is welcomed will foster better patient care. Nicholls et al. (1996) suggested that each float nurse and each unlicensed assistive personnel (UAP) being pulled into a different work unit be assigned an available resource person to maintain a continued level of acceptable patient care.

The third staffing issue to be considered is the use of agency personnel to maintain adequate unit staffing levels. Institutions are now being held liable under the principle of "apparent agency" (Guido, 1997). When patients cannot differentiate between employment of a nurse by the hospital (facility) and that by a different outside agency, the law often will conclude that the agency nurse is to be treated as an employee of the institution for the "purpose of corporate and vicarious liability" (Guido, 1997, p. 282). Therefore, managers must be aware of the skills, knowledge, and abilities of agency nurses they employ so as to maintain adequate patient care and safety. Requiring an orientation and maintaining a background information sheet on each agency nurse can potentially minimize application of the Ostensible/Apparent Agency Doctrine. This doctrine is not described here, but the implications of the agency nurse as relief are discussed.

Most independent agencies that supply temporary contract nursing services to health care settings will screen applicants for levels of skills and experience in bedside nursing. A variety of examinations may be given to ensure that the temporary staff nurse is familiar with medications frequently administered on services that are approved for an assignment. The agency may keep a record of skills that the nurse claims to possess (to the agency interviewer) or particular modes of patient care that the nurse has performed independently and successfully. However, these records rarely are transmitted to the temporary job site or to the employing health facility.

DOCUMENTATION OF SKILLS FOR
TEMPORARY OR AGENCY NURSES

The temporary or as-needed (PRN) nurse or a relief staff nurse from a private agency should maintain a portfolio containing a checklist of skills and personal experience. The documentation within the portfolio can serve as a continuing record for the temporary/relief nurse to carry to job assignments to validate as appropriate a patient care assignment. A copy of the skills list can be sent to health care facilities when they request additional temporary staff nurse assistance. Such lists can be used to determine the best placement for the PRN or relief nurse within the facility. If a PRN or relief nurse frequently is assigned to the same unit, then the skills list can be reviewed by the nurse manager on that unit to determine any limitations on patient assignments for that specific individual.

DELEGATION AND THE STAFF NURSE

The maximization of all employees' skills in today's health care delivery system requires proper delegation of duties to deliver safe and competent care to every patient. Delegation is defined by the National Council of State Boards of Nursing (NCSBN, 1995) as "transferring to a competent individual the authority to perform a selected nursing task in a selected situation. The nurse retains accountability for the delegation" (p. 2). At the staff nurse level, delegating and directing patient care is a demanding job. In 1995, the NCSBN allowed RNs to "delegate certain nursing tasks to [LPNs]/licensed vocational nurses [LVNs] and [UAPs]" (p. 2). It is important that the nurse in charge of delegating duties maintains responsibility to see that those duties are carried out within the standards of practice and according to the institution's policies and procedures. It is likewise important that the nurse understands that personal accountability is retained for the assessment of the patient's needs/circumstances and the delegation of tasks to other health care providers.

The RN is legally responsible to know the expected level of competency that an LPN/LVN or a UAP possesses and the ability to carry out the task delegated. The LPN/LVN or UAP under the RN's direction is held accountable both for his or her acceptance of the delegated task and for the way in which the task is carried out (NCSBN, 1995).

RNs are accountable for following the laws that govern their practice. They might be unclear as to what or when they can delegate. To properly delegate any task, the RN will need to follow an assessment protocol for the situation at that time. According to Huber (1996), five questions need to be considered prior to delegating tasks to others. Table 9.2 identifies those questions.

TABLE 9.2   Questions to Ask When Delegating

1. Is there potential harm in delegating a task?
2. Is the task to be delegated too complex for the delegatee to handle?
3. Does the delegatee have the ability to problem solve?
4. Is the outcome of the task predictable?
5. Does the delegatee have the skills necessary to interact with the client adequately to carry out the task?

SOURCE: Adapted from Huber (1996).

Good communication is imperative for the success of the task delegated; therefore, directions need to be clearly stated (Hansen and Washburn, 1992). Supervision of the task delegated also is considered part of the nurse's role. Professional issues in the nursing process such as assessment and evaluation should not be delegated; tasks and procedures may be delegated. The use of professional judgment by the RN is expected under nursing standards of care and cannot be delegated (Huber, 1996).

The nurse must be aware of the ability levels of each member of the staff who may receive delegated assignments. Schwartz (1992) identified five rules of delegation that answer the question, "Is this the right person for the task?" Table 9.3 identifies those questions.

The use of nurse extenders or UAPs is intertwined with the issue of delegation and supervision by a nurse. As noted earlier, delegation of tasks can be made to individuals from LPNs/LVNs to UAPs who have limited or relatively brief formalized health care education. An organization that is using more and more UAPs will have to be responsible for hiring, orienting, and training those individuals. The nurses who take on the major responsibility for patient care will be supervising them. Nurses always must keep in mind the needs and safety of the patient. What is "right for the patient" must be kept in the forefront of the delegating process.

Another issue in the delegation process is the leadership ability of the RN in charge of delegation of tasks. Use of Benner's theory of practice suggests that different nurses may delegate tasks differently, based on the level of experience of the nurse delegator (Bostrom and Suter, 1992). The survey conducted by Bostrom and Suter (1992) demonstrated that nurses with more experience in clinical practice evaluated a broader range of factors in making assignments and delegating tasks than did those with lesser experience. Nurses must be brought up to a level of delegation ability that fosters success before they can feel confident in the delegation process. Facilities should provide a mentorship program to nurture the skills of nurses who seek greater responsibility in overseeing the process of delegation.

TABLE 9.3 Five Rules of Delegation

1. The person is available to receive the delegated assignment.
2. Ability of the delegatee is sufficient to perform the assigned task.
3. Do not overburden one employee with an overwhelming task.
4. Save delegated tasks for employees with seniority rather than assigning new employees unfamiliar tasks.
5. Consider the time and complexity of the task and delegate the correct number of personnel required to successfully perform the skill in a timely manner.

SOURCE: Adapted from Schwartz (1992).

DOCUMENTATION OF SKILLS FOR EVALUATION AND DELEGATION

Registered nurses are evaluated periodically according to institutional policies. In an acute care facility, the nurse manager of the unit to which a nurse is regularly assigned normally presents the performance evaluation. Documentation of anecdotal events that are obtained on a predetermined day by the manager or assessment designee can be useful in providing a snapshot of performance. When the snapshot information is added to any unusual events that are acknowledged by patients, family members, or peers, the accuracy of the performance evaluation is improved. This system of collecting performance information can serve as objective anecdotal documentation for purposes of evaluation. The evaluator should guard against the "halo effect" of an unusual event becoming the standard and not the exception. An evaluation should reflect the average or usual performance with mention of outstanding single experiences supporting professional growth.

The written evaluation should contain a skills and experience checklist that can be updated with each evaluation period. It is this skills and experience checklist that can assist the nurse in delegating special patient assignments. Although time does not permit a review of all the staff nurse's skills checklist every 8 or 12 hours at the beginning of a tour of duty, a staff list with an alphabetical or numerical designation for differing skills and experiences can be reviewed at a glance during the task of delegating patient assignments.

Delegation of starting or continuing intravenous (IV) solutions to the LPN/LVN is governed by the various states' nurse practice acts. In some states, IV certification must be completed following the formal educational program for the LPN/LVN. Where an LPN/LVN cannot perform IV skills, an RN must be assigned to cover for that particular skill as part of their patient assignments. This possible skills gap must be explored when floating or pulling of LPNs/LVNs may occur. The RN's workload needs to be examined when the temporary/relief nurse is limited in skills that are necessary for specifically assigned patients. An acceptable acuity distribution of patients will provide the best possible expectation of patient care by similarly skilled nurses. When an experienced nurse is overloaded due to less experienced or unfamiliar staff members, patient safety and standards of care can be jeopardized.

In-service education departments within health care facilities usually maintain information regarding the skills and continuing education levels of nurses and UAPs. This information should be available to the nursing manager at the time of employment and as additions to each individual's records are made.

The process of adding and maintaining the documentation of skills and experience should rest with the individual health caregiver (LPN/LVN or UAP). When this checklist of abilities is required at the onset of employment and is updated on a prescribed timetable, accurate and timely information will be available to the nurse making patient care delegation decisions.

CONCLUSION

Although no absolute staffing ratio can be predetermined based on the constantly changing patient mix, acuity, and influx of admissions, the RN needs to be on vigil for the safety and well-being of assigned patients. When staffing is determined to be less than adequate, reporting the situation to the next person in the chain of command is highly recommended. Experienced nursing supervisors can help in the decision making to seek additional staff if that is determined to be necessary. If questions related to safe patient care remain, then documentation of the circumstances is appropriate. Any written reports of concern need to be passed along to nursing administration for review. The nurse should remember the issue of patient abandonment and remain on duty to provide the best care that is possible under the circumstances.

Delegation to UAPs or to newly licensed staff members must be made with the patient acuity in mind. Backup assessment and assistance from more experienced LPNs/LVNs is an alternative. Patient care assignments should reflect attention to the patients' needs and level of care necessary, with knowledge of the education, skills, and experience of staff members.

CASE STUDY

Ms. K was involved in an automobile accident resulting in a bruised head, a possible concussion, and a deep laceration to her right knee. She was taken to the local hospital and was referred by her physician to an orthopedist. Ms. K did not have any fractures. She was observed for possible head injury and treated for pain while continuing to be hospitalized. Over the next several days, Ms. K complained of increasing pain in her right leg, especially over the knee. She was persistent with calling for the nurses over the room voice call system. She told the new physician about her pain. She refused to have the bed sheet placed on top of her right leg because the weight of the sheet sent shooting pain up her leg. Her knee was swollen, was hot to touch, and had turned bright yellow. The orthopedist told her that her leg problems had to run their course, and he did nothing else for her while maintaining her on bed rest in the hospital. She had attempted to contact her family but could not reach her family members by phone. She asked the nurses to help her contact them but was dismissed as a complainer. During one episode, she was very loud and angry at the nurse who would not help her get in touch with her family. The nurse reported and recorded that Ms. K was confused and hallucinating.

Two separate issues evolved within the next few days. Ms. K's family found her and began to be her advocate, and the orthopedist brought in another orthopedist, who diagnosed fulminating necrotizing fascitis from staphylococcus and streptococcus infection. She underwent extensive surgery to drain multiple abscesses in the tissue around the bone.

Ms. K filed a lawsuit against the hospital, nurses, and first physician. She claimed false imprisonment by the nurses based on their refusal to aid her in contacting her family when she was unable to help herself. She also lodged claims of failure to provide an ongoing assessment of her complaints of knee pain and failure to follow up on the physical findings of her knee.

The nurse's actions were found to meet the legal definition for false imprisonment. Furthermore, the nurse failed to properly assess the patient's condition. If the physician failed to respond to the nurse's request for a physician assessment of the leg, due to continuous and increasing signs of infection, then the proper action would have been to report the situation to nursing administration. All facts should have been carefully recorded in the medical record without personal comments or bias statements related to the physician response.

RECORDING PATIENT CARE IN THE EMERGENCY DEPARTMENT

10

Sue E. Meiner

Chapter Outline

As the specialty of emergency nursing has evolved over the past 30 years, the role of the emergency nurse (EN) has evolved into a role with expanded responsibilities to recognize and evaluate emergent and critical conditions. The process of triage, used on the battlefield and in large-scale disasters, became the normal action in the emergency room, now referred to as the emergency department (ED). This refined practice of triage is used to separate patients with the most serious and life-threatening conditions from patients with minor, non-life-threatening conditions. Whereas care is given to the breadth of conditions presented, the methodology for providing that treatment is delivered following detailed guidelines and approaches.

According to the Emergency Nurses Association (1991a), every patient entering the emergency care system is to be assessed to determine priorities of care based on a set of needs. These include physical, psychological, and social needs. Other considerations include the internal organized flow of the ED. After the priority of meeting health needs, administrative needs are considered in the overall functioning of the ED.

Discussion is confined to common problems seen in the ED, areas of highest occurrence in litigation claims, in-hospital triage, and the responsibilities of the EN for documenting patient management. These responsibilities cannot be separated from the guidelines established in the ED for expediting interventions, life support, and other treatments.

LITIGATION FINDINGS IN THE EMERGENCY DEPARTMENT

Instances of not meeting the standards of care in the ED were reported by Beckmann (1996). She analyzed malpractice cases in the hospital setting. In the database used, she found that 9.37% of the 747 nursing malpractice cases recorded identified the ED as the area in which adverse nursing-based outcomes occurred.

The predominant departure from the standard of emergency nursing care was in the area of inadequate communication with other health care team members. According to Beckmann, the other areas identified, in order of number of negligence claims, were as follows:

- Medication administration errors
- Environmental safety negligence
- Nursing negligence associated with inadequate physician care
- Nursing intervention negligence

Details regarding medication administration errors were discussed in Chapters 4 and 5.

COMMONLY ENCOUNTERED EMERGENCY DEPARTMENT PATIENT PROBLEMS

When the statistics regarding common patient problems associated with adverse outcomes were examined, Beckmann (1996) listed the following health problems in order of number of occurrences:

1. Pregnancy-related complications
2. Nervous system disorders
3. Gastrointestinal tract problems
4. Respiratory conditions

5. Less statistically significant conditions
    A. Cardiovascular conditions
    B. Wounds with or without infection
    C. Musculoskeletal alterations
    D. Multiple trauma
    E. All other diverse categories

When patients enter the ED for treatment of these health complaints, the coordination of care requires appropriate communication among the health care team members. When adverse outcomes were reviewed by Beckmann (1996), she found that the most frequent adverse outcomes were caused by poor or inadequate communication among the team members. The most striking area was with nurses failing to inform the physician of abnormal assessment data or failing to communicate that the patient's condition has not improved prior to discharge from the ED. These problems of communication include failing to record data and failing to read data that are recorded by each member of the ED.

CONSENT ISSUES IN THE EMERGENCY DEPARTMENT

An emergency doctrine of consent is in place when interventions are needed to sustain life and prevent additional damage. Consent can be obtained after treatment is rendered (Meisel and Kuczewski, 1996). In the case of an intoxicated trauma victim, consent is implied if cooperation is present. However, an intoxicated patient's signed consent is invalid (Lanros and Barber, 1997).

Nurses in the ED often are involved in obtaining blood specimens for alcohol levels. The laws vary from state to state, but the following guidelines are recommended by Lanros and Barber (1997). Passive consent is adequate if the patient presents an arm for the venipuncture. When a legal warrant to draw the blood specimen is present and is accompanied by the police, a specimen can be obtained if the patient is cooperative. However, when no warrant is presented and the patient refuses to voluntarily have the venipuncture, then the nurse should not attempt a blood draw. This situation should be returned to the physician or ED manager for resolution.

EMERGENCY NURSING SKILLS

Facione and Facione (1996) found that the EN must have essential critical thinking skills that include interpretation, analysis, evaluation, inference, explanation, and self-correction. The quality of documentation is firmly based on critical thinking, which is transferred to the written or computerized emergency record. The EN must demonstrate knowledge of advanced technology coupled with high-level clinical analysis and judgment.

EMERGENCY DEPARTMENT TRIAGE

Lanros and Barber (1997) discussed the advantages of having a nurse triage system in place in the ED. In their discussion of these benefits, they stated, "A nurse, with responsibility for making rapid decisions based on speedy but accurate assessment of each patient who presents, decid[es] who needs immediate intervention and where, and who can tolerate a short wait" (p. 6). This system of rapid, systematic collection of data related to the patient's chief complaint is recorded in a succinct and complete manner, and the patient is referred onto the level of care determined by the assessment. The acuity of the patient's needs determines the appropriate interventions and, therefore, the appropriate patient area for needed care. Triage is done in a collaborative effort to ensure timely patient care.

When the flow of patients and services pivots around decisions made by the EN, any departure from the standards of care can cause serious problems for all other members of the emergency team. Patient records need established review to determine consistency with the triage protocols.

EMERGENCY NURSING ASSESSMENT
AND COMMUNICATION

Nurses must assess each patient using the parameters of physical, psychosocial, and holistic information based on subjective and objective findings. Recording observations, physical assessment findings, and responses to treatments and medications, as well as frequently analyzing the results of multiple laboratory values, never can become routine. Communicating abnormal findings to the appropriate member of the health care team is an area that has been identified as problematic. Beckmann (1996) found that failure to notify the physician regarding a patient's unimproved condition prior to discharge was high on the list of liability issues in emergency nursing practice. The seriousness associated with a delay in appropriate treatment, as the result of poor or incomplete communication, often led to lengthier readmissions or even the deaths of patients.

When problems were connected to nursing assessment and observation, data indicated that omission of these activities was more responsible than improperly performed assessments and observations. The taking of vital signs after the initial admission procedure was found to be lacking in many cases, including those where the initial readings were abnormal. Other areas included a failure to monitor adequate urinary output. When an indwelling urinary catheter was not in place, measuring urinary elimination often was omitted from the ongoing assessment.

RECORDING ADMINISTRATION OF CONSCIOUS SEDATION

Conscious sedation is given during a variety of painful procedures done in emergency situations. Conscious sedation renders the patient vulnerable to harm from the loss of protective reflexes. The EN must be knowledgeable in all aspects of administration, monitoring, and emergent response to reverse the effect of the drugs if an untoward reaction develops.

Recording the exact drug, dosage, time, route of administration, and patient response is essential. Continuous monitoring until the protective reflexes return is vital to prevent complications that can include respiratory arrest. Caution is needed in the administration of conscious sedation with infants and young children.

Emergency procedures and equipment should be reviewed periodically, and forms should be maintained regarding the attendance and successful performance of resuscitation by antidote and adjuvant treatment. Records related to in-service classes need to be reviewed throughout the year to ensure the safety of ED patients.

USING FLOW SHEETS IN THE EMERGENCY DEPARTMENT

The flow sheet format frequently is used in the ED to record care given including nursing assessment and response. This checkoff charting format should be accompanied by areas for recording the critical thinking elements required of the EN. When these are not present or are not used, communication among health care team members can easily be lost.

RECORDING CRITICAL THINKING IN THE EMERGENCY DEPARTMENT

Recording critical thinking associated with performance of nursing interventions can be difficult when the form has limited space for narrative comments. Succinct technical writing is needed to record critical thinking evaluations that could affect care outcomes. The ED nurse must anticipate appropriate responses or interventions while understanding the rationale behind the interventions. Eliminating extraneous words while succinctly recording the facts can be challenging. Eggland (1997) referred to the quality of documentation as resting on the ability to explicitly inform others of the nature of care given.

Many ED flow sheets include spaces or boxes for the dates and times when specific nursing interventions are completed. According to defined standards of care, it is necessary to document additional information to demonstrate critical thinking. Laboratory data can be a significant component in assessing the emergency patient's condition. Recording the time that specimens are collected, the time that a report is received, and any resulting communication of the findings to the emergency room physician or private physician is essential. When information is obtained from another health team member, a name or initials of the person can be helpful if additional information related to the report is needed.

Physicians' orders often are placed in one area of a single-page ED record. When this is the format used, marks made to identify an order that has been carried out frequently are obscured. This can pose a problem when more than one nurse is responding to the orders. In this circumstance, communication is vital to the safety of the patient.

RECORDING PRE-HOSPITAL INFORMATION

Documentation of the signs and symptoms that led to the need for an emergency visit is important. Obtaining pre-hospital data using a primary source of information is preferred to secondary or hearsay sources. However, in trauma situations resulting from accidents, emergency technicians or paramedics are the only source of information available until family members can be located. As soon as possible, secondary sources of information need to be reached to determine the pre-accident health and mental status of the patient.

When the emergency personnel give the verbal report of vital signs and status of injuries, attention needs to be given to this report so as to compare the pre-hospital findings to the initial assessment in the ED. The ambulance report form will have the patient's status recorded for review later as events are being recorded surrounding the ED care given. This report is important to scan, to determine that all of the information was given, and to locate the next of kin to obtain additional information.

Urdan, Davie, and Thelan (1992) identified a strong correlation between the time required for definitive therapy for an injury to be initiated and the outcome. Mortality is a direct result of untimely intervention.

RECORDING EMERGENCY DEPARTMENT INFORMATION

Once any action is taken in the ED, the care has switched from the responsibility of the emergency personnel to that of the ED personnel. The exact time of the transfer of responsibility needs to be recorded on the ED record. Other information that must be recorded as soon as an action is taken includes the treatment that was given, the rationale for the treatment decision, and communication with other health team members, especially any physician involved with treatment decisions.

When more than one physician is directing care and giving verbal orders for emergency treatments, care must be taken to record the correct orders from the physician giving those orders. In the fast-paced environment of a busy ED, keeping track of orders can be quite challenging. The potential exists for a written order to be carried out after it was already completed due to an earlier verbal order. If the verbal order is written and a notation is made that it was completed, then this duplication of treatment can be avoided.

When an EN administers an emergency medication following ED protocols, the medical record should contain details of the assessment, decision making, and actions taken with regard to the medication. These actions will require the cosignature of a physician unless the actions are covered by the state's advanced practice nursing certification.

ALTERED STATES OF CONSCIOUSNESS

Assessing the level of consciousness (LOC) in the ED is a common activity. Trauma victims often have head injuries that require consistent vigilance. This is the highest priority of assessment on a neurologically impaired patient without life-threatening injuries. Verbal arousal of a patient is the initial stimulus for the LOC assessment. The charting of findings from assessment of arousal behaviors can be ambiguous. Lanros and Barber (1997) recommended avoiding words that can be difficult to interpret such as "lethargic," "stuporous," and "obtunded." Objective descriptions of the response to assessments of arousal should be recorded in the medical record. Objective terms such as "slurred speech," "unable to keep eyes open," and "speech trails off prior to completing a verbal response" should be used. Assessments comprise multiple areas of focus. The examinations of reflexes, extremity strength and sensation, and motor activities are also components of a neurological assessment. Eye signs are important to include in an examination for LOC. Table 10.1 provides various eye assessments related to LOC.

TABLE 10.1 Eye Assessment for Level of Consciousness Evaluation

Abnormal eye movements	Not to be tested in conscious patients
Doll's eye reflex	Eyes move in the same direction as the head
Extraocular movement	Examined for PERLA (*p*upils, *e*qual, *r*eact to *l*ight and *a*ccommodation)
Eye signs	Alterations in pupillary size and reactivity
Pupils	Examined for size, shape, and abnormal findings

TABLE 10.2 Conditions of Patients in Which the Glasgow Coma Scale Is Ineffective

1. The presence of an endotracheal tube
2. Limb fractures or severe injury
3. The patient speaks a foreign language
4. The patient is profoundly deaf
5. The patient is under the influence of drugs or alcohol
6. Modification is required for use with neonates and children

SOURCE: Adapted from Lanros and Barber (1997).

Using a specific diagnostic tool that can provide a quantitative measurement of a patient's neurological status is highly recommended in the ED. The most commonly used tool to assess neurological state is the Glasgow Coma Scale (GCS). Numbers are obtained from scoring three factors with a maximum healthy score of 15. These factors are eye opening, best verbal response, and best motor response. If the GCS is the preferred tool, then some patients will score poorly. Table 10.2 provides conditions of patients that preclude the use of the GCS. When the GCS cannot be used effectively, recording objective data is necessary.

The EN must have sound critical judgment in assessing the difference between a coma resulting from neurological insult and one that is metabolic in origin. The difference often is hard to establish. The most reliable clue is the eye response to light stimuli. In a metabolic coma, a light reflex usually will occur unless eye disease or trauma is present. Assessing a respiratory pattern of Kussmaul (rapid and deep) breathing will provide additional data to identify severe acidosis related to a metabolic disorder instead of a neurological alteration.

ENVIRONMENTAL SAFETY NEGLIGENCE

Patients that are in the ED experience periods of intense activity with periods of observation and minimal patient-focused activity. Often, these variations occur while results from tests are pending or staff members are waiting for a response from a consultant on a specialized case. Adverse outcomes associated with environmental safety issues are associated mainly with falls. The breach of standards of care where falls are involved includes failing to assist a patient getting off a stretcher, failing to assist after a complaint of dizziness, failing to use side rails on a stretcher, and leaving the patient unattended. Other areas of environmental safety include raising side rails without securing extremities that might become caught and injured in the mechanism.

The adverse outcomes resulting from these negligent occurrences include simple to compound fractures, sprains, superficial and deep lacerations, and a unilateral loss of sight. These adverse outcomes could be prevented in most instances. Ongoing assessment and observation accompanied by open communication with the patient might prevent these occurrences.

NURSING NEGLIGENCE ASSOCIATED WITH INADEQUATE PHYSICIAN CARE

The main finding in this category is a failure to obtain assistance for a patient when the responding physician is found to have given inadequate medical care, attention, and follow-up to a patient. The determination of inadequate medical care, attention, and follow-up is within the EN's responsibility as a patient advocate. It can be exemplified by not being able to perform a procedure, ignoring nursing assessment findings that are crucial to care decisions, and planning a discharge when the patient's condition is unstable.

In any of these circumstances, the recommended action of the EN is to contact the immediate nursing supervisor for assistance in getting a response from the original physician or for assistance in finding another physician to care for the patient. Recording the facts of these situations without placing blame or criticizing in any manner is considered to be meeting the risk management obligation of the EN. The facts can include contacting a nursing supervisor, calling a physician with a patient status report, receiving orders, and the normal charting associated with the nursing process.

PREPARATION THROUGH CONTINUING EDUCATION

ED priorities include a rapid, focused assessment with carefully understood interventions. ENs will benefit by additional preparation to meet the standards of the emergency nursing practice.

Courses that can prepare the EN for the expected rapid, prioritized response to trauma or health emergencies include Advanced Cardiac Life Support and Advanced Trauma Life Support as well as the Trauma Nurse Core Course. Often, a facility designated as a "Trauma I" facility will offer continuing education courses by the physicians for nurses, paramedics, and emergency medical technicians.

CONCLUSION

The documentation of nursing care given to patients in the ED presents many challenges. Critical thinking, using emergency standard protocols, and maintaining solid communications are essential to this specialty. In addition, prioritization or performing triage of patients can pose a unique opportunity for ED nurses in the area of documentation. In the evolving practice of charting by exception, it is essential to scrutinize documentation to ensure that standards are met, critical thinking is clearly evident, and communication is complete.

CASE STUDY

Mr. A, a 45-year-old married man and the father of five children, was admitted to the ED via ambulance in an unresponsive state. His wife accompanied him in the ambulance. During the initial interview with the wife, it was learned that the only recent health deviation was an infected root canal procedure that was being treated with antibiotics. Several orders were written on the chart by the admitting physician. The nurse took an initial set of vital signs that included a temperature of 101°F, a pulse rate of 110, and a respiratory rate of 28 with deep excursions noted. The blood pressure was 130/88. No other vital signs were taken for the remainder of the patient's 3-hour stay in the ED.

Dextrose 5% in water was the intravenous fluid administered. When a finger stick for blood glucose indicated a reading of "HHH" on the monitor, the nurse reported the meter as defective and ordered another one from the laboratory.

An hour after admission, no appreciable change in the patient's condition had occurred, and the wife asked the nurse to have a physician come to see her husband. The nurse informed the physician of the wife's concerns. The physician returned to the room and told the wife that he would not be sure of a diagnosis until the laboratory results were back. The wife remained next to the stretcher in a fully curtained cubicle.

The nurse called the lab for the results of the tests, as requested by the physician. She was told that the tests were being analyzed again because an abnormal finding was recorded. Another 15 minutes go by before the lab calls the unit secretary with the results of a blood glucose of 1,200 mg/dl with two retests. The secretary recorded this information on the lab report clipboard at the main ED desk and highlighted it in pink.

Several minutes later, the wife yelled for help. The nurse and physician came into the room and found the patient in full arrest. After multiple attempts to resuscitate, the patient was pronounced dead.

In this case, the ED team was not a team. Each member worked independently of the others with a lack of direct or indirect communication. The nurse failed to complete an assessment of an undiagnosed diabetic in a state of metabolic acidosis with an extremely high blood glucose level. Only a few of the breaches of standards of nursing care will be identified. These include failure to follow up on abnormal vital signs, failure to follow physician orders for finger stick blood glucose, and failure to recognize a normal result from a piece of equipment that is to be used by trained and evaluated personnel only. They also include failure to follow up on laboratory data and failure to communicate with the physician concerning an abnormal lab finding prior to an official report.

The nurse was not alone in liability. The hospital, ED physician, lab staff member, and nurse all were named in this claim of wrongful death. The award was $3,000,000.

RECORDING PATIENT CARE IN THE CRITICAL CARE UNIT

11

Sue E. Meiner

Chapter Outline

The varied roles of the nurse in the critical care area often are dominated by technical equipment. An understanding and efficient use of these highly complex biomedical machines is a requirement that may overshadow direct patient care. The ability to monitor patient care with machines while administering quality nursing care is a challenge for the critical care (CC) nurse.

The charting systems used often are developed by the individual facility to meet the needs of medical and nursing staff. If these charting systems are carefully developed, then the medical record can reflect a thorough accounting of the care given and the patient response to that care. However, this is an area with great responsibility for life-and-death attention that may or may not be associated with the biomedical component of care in a technologically advanced CC unit.

The variety of CC units can include the medical CC unit, surgical CC and trauma units, and the coronary care unit that was one of the earliest specialty care areas. No differentiation is attempted to separate the unique aspects of the wide variety of CC units. Basic areas that have been linked to litigation have been selected for the focus. Although not exhaustive in CC practices, this chapter presents information related to specific issues and the related documentation needs that face nurses working in the general CC unit.

LITIGATION FINDINGS
IN CRITICAL CARE NURSING

Beckmann (1996) found specific areas of nursing practice that were the central elements in litigation. Among them were inadequate communication with the physician regarding information from the nursing assessment, negligent nursing assessment (primarily from omission), and mistakes in the administration of medications (see Chapters 4 and 5). Communication, nursing assessment, and medication administration are the foundations of nursing practice as well as documentation of outcomes.

ETHICAL DILEMMAS IN
THE CRITICAL CARE UNIT

Decisions made by primary care providers usually are given to the CC nurse to implement. The CC nurse often is confronted with issues that may test ethical and moral concerns. These concerns surround the dilemma of maintaining life at all costs and efforts when no quality of life is possible (Urden, Davie, and Thelan, 1992). The quality of life issue has replaced the total and absolute sanctity of maintaining life even on support equipment for as long as necessary until life cannot be sustained by the human body. "Technology encourages death to be viewed as a symptom to be treated, not as a life event," (Urden et al., 1992, p. 18).

The CC nurse must face ethical decisions while providing quality nursing care in a highly technological environment that often seems too clinical. The art of the CC nurse in providing compassionate care often is missing from the record of care given. This qualitative measure of compassion and advocacy never should be dismissed during adversarial litigation proceedings. The standards of routine practice in the use of biomedical devices can be used as the yardstick for measuring the quality of care.

MONITORING AND RECORDING
THE ELECTROCARDIOGRAPH

The most common type of biomedical equipment used in CC units is the continuous electrocardiograph. The use of this device has been extremely beneficial to patients with cardiac problems that require the most rapid response to changes. These changes can have life-or-death results if emergency interventions are not initiated as soon as the irregularities of a cardiac pattern are identified by the CC nurse or the monitor technician assisting in the observation of the patient.

The advanced knowledge and skill needed to perform cardiac monitoring and charting behaviors in the CC unit require many hours of additional nursing education and evaluation of proficiency. This proficiency needs to be documented in the personnel records of CC nurses and with the nursing supervisor in immediate line of authority. Renewals of proficiency should be monitored by the supervisor in charge of the nursing personnel. This check and balance can prevent outdated knowledge of cardiac emergency treatments from being practiced.

Charting Routine Nursing Care of the Monitored Patient

When the electrocardiograph electrodes are being prepared for attachment to the patient, care needs to be taken to secure the connection properly. The flow sheet should have an area to record the following information:

1. The patient is instructed in rationale and method of monitoring.
2. The chest wall is prepared for electrode placement.
3. The cardiac monitor is adjusted to obtain a viewable complex.
4. Alarms are set for high and low parameters of the heart rate.
5. Alarms are set for audibility of the monitoring nurse or technician.
6. Initial recording of the cardiac rhythm is placed in the record.

The cardiac conduction pathway is recorded on the electrocardiograph. The proper preparation and administration of the electrodes is essential in the recognition of abnormalities in the cardiac pattern. At least one printout of that pattern must be done to ensure that the procedure has been proficiently completed. Thereafter, the printouts are required at regular intervals for unchanged patterns or when any pathological change occurs in the patient's baseline.

Charting Abnormal Cardiac Rhythms

Interpretation of the cardiac rhythm is a skill that must be practiced regularly. A systematic method incorporates a basic six-step process (Table 11.1). When the cardiac rhythm has been determined, it must be compared to the previous reading for changes as well as the baseline reading obtained on admission. When changes are identified that show continued or new pathology in the pattern, the

TABLE 11.1 One System for Interpretation of an Electrocardiograph

1. Measure the rates of the atrial and ventricular beats
2. Analyze the R-R interval
3. Analyze the P waves
4. Measure the P-R interval
5. Examine the P and the Q-R-S complex to determine uniformity
6. Analyze the Q-R-S complex

physician of record must be informed. If the change is a life-threatening one, then the unit protocol usually will call for the CC physician or resident physician on call to come to the unit immediately.

CHARTING DURING A CARDIAC AND/OR RESPIRATORY EMERGENCY

The term "code blue" has been used in hospital settings for many decades. This term is used as the emergency call in life-threatening situations. The call is intended to alert a specially trained team to respond immediately. When it is announced over a public address system, team members may be called from a variety of service units to the location of the emergency. Larger CC units might have an internal alarm system that is not broadcast throughout the entire building. When this is the case, all members of the code team are internal to the CC unit and are not needed from other areas of the building.

A set of forms is placed on the mobile cart that contains nearly all emergency lifesaving medications, equipment, and sterile trays with lifesaving procedure instruments. This cart is referred to as the "crash cart." The forms include the advanced cardiac life support algorithms and flow sheets for recording time, actions, personnel, medications, procedures, and end of code disposition and status of the patient. Some facilities might use more than one form or flow sheet to record this information. Table 11.2 provides an example of a blank code record form. A member of the code team should serve as a recorder of times, actions, medications, and personnel in attendance. The form becomes a part of the patient's permanent record and may be vital to litigation to prove the sequence of emergency interventions.

CRITICAL CARE FLOW SHEETS

CC flow sheets were developed to assist nurses in minimizing the amount of time spent on recording care so as to permit maximal time in patient care and support.

Table 11.2 Example of a Code Record Form

CODE BLUE RECORD: page # ___ of ___.‖ ___ Cardiac; ___ respiratory; ___ other
Patient Name: _____ Room: _____ Date: _____
Time Initiated: _____ ; CPR Team: (names & credentials) _____
_____

Vital Signs		Medications		Actions Taken	Laboratory	
Time	Reading	Bolus	I.V.		ABGs	other

Time	Notes/Actions

End of Code Time: _____ ; Status after Code: _____

Disposition: Special Unit: ___; Morgue: ___; Other: ___. Code Director: _____

Recorder: _____ ; Nurse: _____ ; others: _____

With the increase in charting content within the CC unit, the flow sheet has proved to be an efficient charting format for recording 24 hours of patient data. Problems with CC forms were discussed in Chapter 4.

Most CC units use a variety of flow sheets to document frequent assessments, interventions, and patient responses to care. Nurses are responsible for the following:

1. Performing a thorough assessment at least every shift
2. Making routine observations
3. Recording biomedical device settings
4. Collecting hemodynamic data
5. Identifying responses to treatments and medications
6. Analyzing the results of all laboratory findings

TABLE 11.3 Essential Critical Care Assessment Items

---

1. Vital signs: temperature, pulse, respiration, and blood pressure (time)
2. Body systems and findings:
   A. Neurological: coma scale, reflexes, limb movement
   B. Cardiovascular: rhythm, regularity, vascular checks, hemodynamics
   C. Respiratory: rate, depth, symmetry, assist device, oxygen saturation[a]
   D. Renal: urine (void, Foley, ostomy), dialysis (abdominal or hemo)[b]
   E. Gastrointestinal: diet (type), appetite (percentage eaten), bowel sounds, date of last bowel movement[c]
   F. Integumentary: skin color, moisture, temperature, condition (staging of pressure ulcers and body chart), edema, treatment, treatment response
3. Pain: quantitative assessment, type, location, treatment, treatment response
4. Tubes: types, drainage
5. Wounds: location, appearance, treatment
6. Intravenous devices: types, location, appearance, site care, tubing change
7. Teaching: patient or named significant other
8. Activities of daily living: bathing, activity, toileting, transfers, eating
9. Laboratory tests and results
10. Procedures performed and patient response
11. Safety: identification, allergy, oxygen setup, suction setup, tongue blade, rails and bed height, alarms set (monitor, ventilator, bed), call light

---

a. Ventilation: endotracheal tube, nasotracheal tube, mode, fraction of inspired oxygen, tidal volume, respiratory rate, positive end expiratory pressure, continuous positive airway pressure, peak inspiratory pressure, treatments.
b. Renal: dialysis, amount in (solution), amount out, balance, cumulative.
c. Gastrointestinal: nasogastric tube residuals.

The flow sheet format facilitates the comparison of previous laboratory findings. Table 11.3 provides a list of basic CC assessment areas.

COMMUNICATING FINDINGS APPROPRIATELY

The communication of abnormal findings to the primary care provider or other health team members is an area that frequently is found to be lacking when medical records are reviewed for litigation purposes. The CC nurse must have knowledge concerning potential reactions to treatment modalities, side effects, interaction or adverse effect of medications, and expected patient responses to treatment. When an untoward or unexpected change occurs with a patient, the information must be communicated to the primary care provider or the physician attending the patient. Critical thinking and decision making are bounded by the scope of practice, with the physician making the patient care decisions in the CC unit. This does not dismiss the nurse from the duty to intervene as a patient advocate (see Chapter 12 for additional information on the duty to intervene).

CRITICAL THINKING IN
CRITICAL CARE

The constant use of critical thinking and decision making in the CC unit is an expectation of the CC nurse. The CC nurse is responsible for maintaining current knowledge of new concepts in disease prevention, pathogenesis, and safe patient care management (Chase, 1997; Darovic, 1995). Continuing education courses or updates to original Advanced Cardiac Life Support or Advanced Trauma Life Support courses are recommended to acquire or maintain appropriate CC nursing skills. These courses prepare the CC nurse for making rapid assessments for prioritizing patient care needs. Documentation of course completion needs to be maintained in the personnel files on the unit for easy review prior to annual performance appraisals or at a designated date once a year.

STANDING ORDERS OR PROTOCOLS
IN THE CRITICAL CARE UNIT

Documentation related to an emergency event must include the immediate treatment given, the rationale for the treatment decision, and all communication between the nurse and the physician and other health team members. Standing physician orders or protocols that reflect current practice standards are commonly used in the CC unit. These are designed to ensure quality patient care in a potential emergency situation where a physician might not be immediately available.

When standing orders or protocols are used in an emergency, specific notations must be made in the medical record. The specific notations must include the date, time, and intervention that was attempted, begun, completed, or omitted. The patient's response (both physical and verbal) and the actions that were taken must be recorded. The names of all individuals associated with the event should be recorded (Kidd and Wagner, 1996).

CONCLUSION

Litigation involving any specialty area evolves around the standards of nursing practice for that specialty, hospital policy and procedures, and generally accepted standards of nursing care. Inadequate nursing assessment, inadequate communication with the physician regarding changes in condition, and medication errors are common to all of these settings and remain the source of most of the malpractice litigation brought against nurses.

CASE STUDY

In the following case, Mrs. B, a 74-year-old woman, was admitted to the CC unit with cardiac arrhythmias and angina. The physician's orders included starting an intravenous (IV) line in a peripheral vein, adding a Heparin solution as a piggybacked IV line, and continuous cardiac monitoring with vital signs every 4 hours. Mrs. B was N.P.O. (nothing by mouth) in preparation for a cardiac catheterization.

Although the monitor alarms were set at a low of 60 beats per minute and a high of 100 beats per minute, the arrhythmia created frequent alarms of brief duration. The primary nurse decided to turn off the alarms while she was charting in front of the monitor in the nurses station.

Another nurse's patient developed asystole (flat line) and stopped breathing. A code blue was called, and Mrs. B's nurse ran to assist in the code, leaving the alarm off.

When the code was stopped, Mrs. B's nurse returned to her charting at the nurse's station. At that time, she noticed that Mrs. B's monitor was recording a bradycardia of 30 beats per minute. As she rushed to the bedside, Mrs. B's heart stopped. All resuscitation efforts failed, and Mrs. B was pronounced dead within 30 minutes.

This case was in litigation for nearly 3 years before a settlement was reached. During that time, the nurse was questioned by multiple management personnel and attorneys, and ultimately she resigned from the hospital. At the time of the deposition, the nurse had no plans of ever continuing in a nursing career. The emotional damage that the nurse suffered had required psychotherapy that was continuing.

The use of biomedical devices must be taken seriously at all times. One careless act of turning off a cardiac monitor alarm led to disastrous results for the patient, the patient's family, the nurse, the nurse's family, the hospital, and the insurance company. A careful understanding of the functioning and purpose of all aspects of equipment used in a patient care area is essential to the health and well-being of the patient. It also is essential to the career well-being of the CC nurse.

RECORDING PATIENT CARE IN THE OBSTETRIC UNIT

12

Sue E. Meiner

Chapter Outline

Many legal hazards face obstetric (OB) nursing personnel. OB nursing also is referred to by other terms such as maternal-newborn, maternity, and perinatal nursing. Most of these terms are interchangeable, with the exception of maternal-newborn. When that term is used, the care of the newborn is included in the role. OB nursing includes care of the mother and the fetus or unborn child throughout the perinatal period. Usually, the care of the newborn does not extend beyond the baby's transfer to the newborn nursery.

The standard of care may be measured and applied by the legal process to examine the behavior and expected performance of OB nursing skills practiced during a specific patient's care. As with other areas of nursing specialty, the performance must meet the average skills practiced by a nurse under similar circumstances. If the care is found to be similar to that of a reasonably prudent nurse with similar background, training, and experience, then the standard of care is met.

LITIGATION FINDINGS IN OBSTETRIC NURSING

Beckmann (1996) found that more than 73% of nursing negligence was charged in response to fetal/newborn injuries and that more than 16% resulted from fetal/newborn deaths (stillborn). The newborn injuries were predominantly brain damage. "The mechanism of injury common to cases of both fetal/newborn injury and fetal/newborn death . . . was failure by the nurse to inform the physician of fetal distress in a timely manner" (p. 206). When the maternal deaths were reviewed, inadequate nursing assessment was identified as the most common reason. All of the maternal deaths were associated with complications of pregnancy prior to admission to the unit, and all mothers were in labor on admission.

The amounts of malpractice payments for maternal injuries ranged from $150,000 to $8,000,000. Fetal/newborn injuries (predominantly brain damage) were compensated in the range of $55,000 to an extreme high of $72,650,000. The basis for many of these decisions by the courts is predicated on verdicts in lawsuits or settlement actions in OB malpractice (Beckmann, 1996).

STANDARDS OF NURSING CARE IN OBSTETRIC NURSING

The nursing profession also determines the standards of care through the standards of nursing education, definition of nursing practice, and establishment of policies and protocols for practice issues. The American Nurses Association and the National League for Nursing set respective standards for practice and education in OB or maternity nursing. Specialty nursing organizations further delineate the specific standards of care to practice within the scope of that specialty.

In OB nursing, the most recognized organization is the Association of Women's Health, Obstetric, and Neonatal Nurses, formerly called the Nurses Association of the American College of Obstetricians and Gynecologists (NAACOG). This organization is willing to disseminate information on standards of care to anyone requesting the literature. Its guidelines often are closely followed in legal actions claiming nursing negligence.

BASIC OBSTETRIC DOCUMENTATION

The standards of OB nursing care contain requirements that the documentation be consistent with the nursing process. Components such as assessment, formulation of nursing diagnoses, planning, intervention, and evaluation are to be used in recording the care of the OB patient and unborn child during the labor and delivery process. Other areas of documentation that are within the standards of care are identification of information and important medical/surgical/OB history of the OB patient. The OB record is specific to the perinatal patient. This record reflects the continuing condition of the mother and fetus. When labor begins, the progress is charted in a manner that is specific for the laboring patient. Recording of changes in the maternal and fetal status includes the rupture of the amniotic membrane and resulting fluid discharge. The type, color, odor, and amount of fluid are required to be recorded. Any medications and intravenous fluids given, as well as any oxygen supplementation, oxytocin augmentation, and treatments or diagnostic tests performed (e.g., ultrasound, pelvimetry), are required to be documented in the labor record.

DYSFUNCTIONAL LABOR RECORDING

Dysfunctional labor can be determined by following the labor progress by means of the Friedman graph (Friedman, 1965). This charting system uses a graph to plot cervical dilatation and degree of descent against lapsed time of labor. When followed by a physical assessment finding that is potentially problematic, a report to the obstetrician is highly recommended. All data collected and physician contact should be recorded in the labor record.

Basic areas of nursing charting remain. These include hourly vital signs with space for additional readings as needed. Additional areas required to be documented include intake and output, mobility or activities, controlled labor methods, patient teaching (e.g., controlled breathing and relaxation), response of the patient to the situation, visitors present, and care given. Visits made by any physicians or other health care providers (e.g., phlebotomist, diagnostic technician, anesthesiologist) are to be noted by time, person, and procedure or reason for the visit. Other notes of importance include those of fetal heart rate (FHR) with pattern descriptors and uterine activity.

FETAL MONITORING

When the use of maternal and fetal electronic monitoring became an expected component of perinatal care throughout the United States, standards were formulated to provide the public with nurses able to recognize and interpret FHR patterns and associated uterine activity. OB nurses are responsible for diagnosing fetal distress during labor with the use of electronic fetal monitoring (EFM), monitoring by auscultation and palpation, or monitoring by manual examination. Table 12.1 displays abbreviations commonly used in charting EFM findings.

Nursing care of the OB patient being monitored by EFM requires that the nurse be knowledgeable regarding the process of labor and delivery, the nursing care needs of laboring women (while providing the fetus with the best opportunity for a safe delivery), and the use of equipment that displays and records the maternal contractions and the FHR pattern.

TABLE 12.1 Common Abbreviations for Charting Electronic Fetal Monitoring Findings

BL	Baseline finding
bpm	Heartbeats per minute
FHR	Fetal heart rate
UC	Uterine contraction
LTV[a]	Long-term variability of fetal heart rate
STV[a]	Short-term variability of fetal heart rate
Late decel	Deceleration in fetal heart rate that appears after the uterine contraction begins and persists after the uterine contraction has ended
Early decel	Deceleration in fetal heart rate that appears anytime between uterine contractions but returns to fetal heart rate baseline prior to the end of the uterine contraction; can resemble a mirror image of the uterine contraction
Var decel	Variable decelerations that do not fit either late or early deceleration patterns
Prolonged decel	Deceleration in fetal heart rate that lasts more than 2 minutes

a. Associated with other subset symbols including +, 0, up arrow, and down arrow.

The nursing assessment of the tracings needs to include baseline variations that can range from 120 to 160 beats per minute. A minimum of 10 minutes is needed prior to determining the baseline range of an FHR. Tachycardia and bradycardia are concerns that require action even if the heart rate returns to the baseline immediately. The action is recording the findings and closely observing for other changes that might indicate fetal distress. Table 12.2 displays common abbreviations of EFM components.

The variability assessment needs to include long-term variability (LTV) and short-term variability (STV). Areas to examine in LTV include amplitude, cyclicity, undulating patterns, and physical findings. Examination of STV is concerned with the presence, absence, or intermittent determination of fetal heart electrical movement from beat to beat milliseconds, as recorded on the tracing.

Actions taken depend on the evaluation of the variability. The possible causes of decreased variability need to be identified. In many instances, the maternal position is changed, maternal oxygen is given, oxytocin is discontinued, and/or tocolytics are given. Even fetal scalp stimulation might be applied to increase the FHR.

Variable decelerations in FHR need further assessment of physical findings to determine the exact pattern of the decelerations. Observation of the FHR on the tracing is essential to differentiate variable decelerations from early or late decelerations. These conditions have extremely different outcomes. Conditions that can cause variable decelerations to occur include umbilical cord compression, decreased umbilical cord perfusion, hypoxia, and a hypercarbic condition.

Early decelerations are associated with fetal head compression during labor or vagal stimulation. The concept of early decelerations is not clearly understood

TABLE 12.2 Common Abbreviations for Electronic Fetal Monitoring Components

EFM	Electronic fetal monitor or monitoring
IUPC	Intrauterine pressure catheter (maternal, internal monitoring)
SE	Spiral electrode (fetal scalp, internal fetal heart rate monitor)
TOCO	Tocodynamometer (maternal, external contraction monitoring)
US	Ultrasonography (external, B-mode for fetal development)

TABLE 12.3 Example of Electronic Fetal Monitoring Documentation of a Single Deceleration

1/12/__	0800	Late decel to 100 bpm × 30 seconds; to BL of 140 bpm after decel; STV +, LTV +

but rarely is nonreassuring. When early decelerations are associated with cephalo-pelvic disproportion in a primigravida, minimal dilation has occurred and the fetus is at a high station (Mattson and Smith, 1993).

Conditions that can be responsible for late decelerations include uteropla-cental insufficiency or an impeded blood flow resulting from a variety of other causes. These causes can include a maternal supine position; uterine hyperstimu-lation; and maternal hypotension from blood loss, medications, anesthesia, or drug abuse. Table 12.3 provides an example of charting a single episode of a late deceleration in the fetal heart as recorded on the EFM tracing.

Documentation Directly on the Fetal Monitor Tracing

The charting of pertinent information on the monitor tracing record is a part of nursing documentation responsibility. Charting maternal position and changes to that position during labor as well as the administration and reason for giving the mother oxygen is vital. All medications given to the mother are recorded on the tracing with the time and administering nurse's signature or initials. All internal examinations with findings of dilatation, station, and effacement are recorded on the tracing. Abnormal findings such as rupture of the membranes (bag of water) and presence of meconium-stained fluid are important to note and report.

LABOR AUGMENTATION WITH OXYTOCIN

When labor augmentation or induction is initiated, exact charting of increases or decreases in oxytocin (Pitocin) infusion is to be placed on the tracing as near to the time of the action as possible. The time and identification of the nurse

TABLE 12.4 Common Indications for Induction or Augmentation of Labor

Maternal	Fetal
1. Chorioamnionitis	1. Fetal death
2. Diabetes	2. Prolonged rupture of membranes
3. History of precipitate labor	3. Postmaturity
4. Slowed progress of labor	4. Rh sensitization

performing the action need to accompany the information placed on the EFM and in the patient's chart.

The goal of administering oxytocin is to mimic natural labor when labor is slowing or is ineffective. The nurse caring for the laboring patient undergoing augmentation must be alert for tetanic contractions and maternal hypotension and must assess for the antidiuretic effect that frequently accompanies oxytocin administration. Each delivery facility has a policy and procedure for administration of intravenous oxytocin. The registered nurse caring for this patient must adhere to the strict guidelines in this policy. Careful charting of the time of each increase or decrease in the dosage, amount of increase or decrease, maternal/fetal assessment prior to each decrease, and full maternal/fetal status immediately after each increase in the dosage is required. The rationale for a decrease must be clearly stated in the record (NAACOG, 1988). Table 12.4 provides influencing factors that are indicators for induction or augmentation of labor with oxytocin.

DELIVERY ROOM DOCUMENTATION

During the second stage of labor (infant delivery) assessment, vigilance and fast-paced responses are necessary. In an uncomplicated delivery, the nurse is responsible for the mother and the newborn's care while the obstetrician and mother complete the birth process. At this time, the documentation is continuous. Maternal and fetal assessment is ongoing. Medications are prepared for the newborn and mother for administration at birth. If any form of anesthesia is being administered, then recording that fact is a necessity. As the newborn is delivered, the exact time is noted; the position of the baby's head at the moment of birth is recorded; and 1-, 5-, and 10-minute postdelivery APGAR scores (a measurement tool to determine newborn well-being) are obtained by the nurse.

The umbilical cord is examined, and the number of vessels is recorded. The lack of one arterial vessel is associated with other anomalies. Blood gases usually are taken, at birth, from the umbilical cord. The nurse must be able to identify the venous vessels from the arterial vessels to properly draw arterial blood gases.

When an episiotomy (perineal incision to facilitate vaginal delivery) is performed, recording the type and anatomical position of the incision is required. Other areas of recording that accompany a normal vaginal delivery are presence and degree of lacerations, assisted delivery with forceps or vacuum pump, and any maternal or fetal side effects resulting from these events (Pillitteri, 1996).

During the third stage of labor, the type of placental delivery is recorded along with any abnormalities in the shape or condition of the placenta. Acknowledgment of the episiotomy closure is recorded. The notation that indicates the transfer of the baby's care to the nursery nurses is followed by the recording of the mother's transfer to the OB recovery room.

DUTY TO INTERVENE

Nurses have an independent duty to intervene if care being given by other health care providers is detrimental to the patient. Physical or emotional injury or other detriment to a patient that is allowed by a nurse's inaction, even though the offending act is done by a physician, can be cause for charges of unprofessional conduct by the nurse licensing boards in various states.

The nurse is an independently licensed health care provider who is required to use a unique body of knowledge to make independent nursing assessments and diagnoses, to implement plans of care, and to evaluate the results of those decisions. Orders from physicians must be reviewed for appropriateness and accuracy prior to implementation. The myth that a nurse must follow physicians' orders exactly as stated or written is regarded as false by both professional nursing organizations and nurse licensing boards.

The professional registered nurse must take full responsibility for the hour-by-hour and day-by-day care of every assigned or contracted patient by observing, reporting, and recording all changes in condition that are significant. When physician intervention is required, the nurse must make every effort to reach the patient's physician in a timely manner. If delays happen, then backup systems need to be in place and periodically rehearsed for those inevitable occurrences.

OB situations often require rapid responses to emergent problems. OB emergencies need to be anticipated, with action plans prepared ahead of time and in-service programs held regularly to review the plans.

When a labor and delivery nurse identifies a deviation from the expected progress for the laboring woman, the physician must be contacted and asked to see the patient in person for a physician's assessment. If the physician does not arrive in a timely manner or fails to respond to the alert, then the nurse continues to be responsible for the well-being of the mother and fetus. The next step is to contact the nurse at the next level of authority.

The nursing departments in hospitals or medical centers with OB services have policies and procedures to follow related to the line of authority and responsibility in crisis situations. The OB nurse should follow his or her agency's policies and guidelines with attention to the duty to intervene when appropriate. If, in the experienced OB nurse's judgment, the primary obstetrician's actions are not appropriate, or if an emergency OB problem is created through inaction, then a plan to enlist a skilled, experienced obstetrician needs to be available. A copy of the American College of Obstetricians and Gynecologists standards and guidelines should be kept on each OB unit. Consulting these guidelines regarding physician behavior and performance can direct nursing responses to perceived problems.

Licensed nurses are responsible for direct and indirect results caused by their actions or inaction. Failure to react to the improper behavior of another health care professional when a patient is injured, or when no action is taken when action is expected, can result in the nurse's being indirectly responsible for injury and/or damages.

CONCLUSION

Although this chapter was not intended to be an exhaustive discussion of all aspects of recording in the OB unit, it represented those areas that are most frequently identified with litigation involving claims of nursing negligence. Nurses employed in OB nursing, especially in the labor and delivery areas, must have expert knowledge of perinatal nursing. Caring for two patients (mother and child) throughout the labor and delivery process is challenging and demands expert-level nursing practice. Subtle changes in maternal or fetal well-being demand immediate responses to achieve a good outcome.

Interpersonal relationships are vital to the teamwork that is needed between the nurse and the physician as well as other health team members. Other professionals include anesthesiologists or anesthetists, ultrasonographers, and laboratory technicians. The failure to communicate with any or all of these health care team members can result in a less than optimal outcome for mother, child, or both.

CASE STUDY

The following case represents the scenario of failure to intervene by reporting a physician problem to the supervising nurse on duty. The physician saw this multigravida (expecting her fourth baby) shortly after admission. She was full-term and determined to be in early labor. Her OB history included a 12-hour first labor, an 8-hour second labor, and a 5-hour third labor. Her children had weighed 6 pounds, 7 pounds 4 ounces, and 7 pounds 6 ounces. The sonogram report from an ultrasound taken the week prior to admission stated that the baby possibly was a macrosomia fetus, estimated at $9\frac{1}{2}$ pounds.

After the physician's examination (dilatation 3 cm, effacement 50%, station –3), oxytocin augmentation was ordered to be given according to written protocol. The physician left the hospital for office hours in a building that adjoined the hospital but required approximately 15 minutes to travel the distance due to elevator use and construction detours.

The oxytocin augmentation was begun according to protocol that called for an increase every 30 to 45 minutes until regular contractions, between 60 and 80 mm mercury, were attained every 2 minutes. After the second increase in oxytocin, the nurse's examination revealed a dilatation of 5 cm, an effacement of 75%, and a station of –3. Following other standing orders of the physician, Demerol (100 mg) was administered by intravenous push. The contractions had not achieved the required regularity or amplitude, so another set of two increases was administered.

After 5 hours, the physician returned to the unit and told the nurse to increase the oxytocin every 15 minutes until contractions were effective. On examination, the patient was at 7 cm and 100% effaced, but the station remained at –3. The FHR began to have repeated variable and early decelerations. The physician ordered an additional increase in the oxytocin, which was performed by the nurse. The FHR began to show late decelerations that returned to the baseline just prior to the next contraction. The nurse recorded these patterns but did not say anything to the physician because the monitor was examined every time that the physician visited the room, which was about every 15 minutes.

After 8 hours, the laboring mother was at 10 cm, completely effaced, but still at station –2. Fundal and supra pubic pressure were ordered by the physician, and the nurse complied. After 30 minutes of pushing, the baby's head was delivered. After multiple maneuvers were attempted (over a 15-minute period) to accomplish delivery, the baby's face was blue, the fetal monitor was in a bradycardia of 30 beats per minute, and the baby was firmly wedged into the pelvis. Although a cesarean birth followed, ultimate brain damage resulted. The settlement was in the neighborhood of $1,800,000 for damages and lifelong care.

This case is an example of following orders without using professional nursing judgment. The registered nurse maintained accurate documentation of the course of events but failed to seek assistance as a patient advocate when the orders and the patient assessment did not follow standards of OB care.

A prudent action would have been to seek assistance from the OB nursing supervisor. This communication with the supervisor could have been done at several times during this unfortunate occurrence. Action was needed when the initial order for oxytocin was given, when the patient failed to progress, and as the oxytocin was continuously being increased without much change in fetal station. The variable decelerations progressed to late decelerations and then bradycardia. By the time fundal and supra pubic pressure were ordered by the physician, whether correctly or incorrectly, the assessment of cephalopelvic disproportion was an all too evident possibility.

RECORDING PATIENT CARE IN THE PEDIATRIC UNIT

13

Sue E. Meiner

Chapter Outline

The pediatric patient often is difficult to assess. Complaints can be vague and quite often are influenced by distraught parents. It is essential for the pediatric nurse to apply the nursing process while thoroughly monitoring the child for abrupt changes in condition or adverse reactions to treatments.

The practice of pediatric nursing involves a wide range of emotion and compassion. Nursing care of children is family nursing with a focus on the immediate need of a child. The emotional impact of a sick child is quite devastating to parents. During this emotion-filled time, instructions for home care are given to the family. Providing a phone number to the parents or guardians of the child for emergency contact in the event of problems or additional questions related to the care of the discharged child is essential for safe and effective follow-up. Documenting these instructions and phone numbers in the medical record, and identifying any materials given to the parents, is a sound practice.

LITIGATION FINDINGS IN PEDIATRIC NURSING

Studies have shown that medication errors and inadequate communication with the physician regarding changes in the child's condition have led to the majority of adverse outcomes in the pediatric patient population. Malpractice awards have ranged from $1,000 to $10,350,000 (Beckmann, 1996).

One legal ramification in pediatric care circumstances is the possibility of a long delay in filing a lawsuit until the child has reached the age of majority. In most states, either an additional 2 years is added to the majority age to cover the normal time period of the statute of limitations or else limitations will not begin to run until the minor has reached a certain age short of adulthood. If the parents file suit on behalf of the minor child, then the settlement or judgment will bar the child from again filing suit for the same cause of action.

PEDIATRIC ASSESSMENT DOCUMENTATION

Assessment of a child is vital to finding a cause for any symptoms that the child is displaying or that the family reports noticing. Assessment in a child requires identifying the level of growth and development as compared to standards in pediatric practice. Because most very young children cannot tell the nurse the exact nature of a problem, some common signs of specific problems are evident. The practitioner with education and experience in pediatrics usually can differentiate common health deviations from subtle signs of developmental abnormalities in a child (Price, 1993).

Charting pediatric assessment must be clear. Avoiding terms such as "normal," "good," "poor," "better," "satisfactory," and "unsatisfactory" should be the standard practice. Descriptions of assessment findings need to be accurate, concise, comprehensive, and objective. Consistently using a sequential manner for recording assessment findings is one preferred way in which to prevent missing an area of assessment documentation that is vital to the ongoing care of the child (Weber and Kelley, 1998).

Family or parent teaching is one of the most important areas for practice and documentation. With the high level of emotion that afflicts the parents of a sick child, instructions for the child's care need to be stated and reinforced with written materials, and follow-up contact by a nurse should be scheduled. All actions need to be recorded in the medical record. Although a flow sheet with simple checkoff boxes might seem like an easy way in which to document parent teaching, a narrative statement with more explicit comments on the material taught and the response of the parents to the instruction is preferred (Ahmann, 1994).

FAULTY COMMUNICATION IN PEDIATRIC NURSING

The second highest area of litigation in pediatric nursing is related to the failure to communicate with the primary health care provider when abnormal assessments are identified. Beckmann (1996) identified specific life-threatening areas of deficits in reporting assessment findings as the "failure to report neurological status changes . . ., circulatory status changes . . ., signs of infection . . ., and neurovascular changes" (p. 191).

Many textbooks, including those on pediatrics, discuss the art of communication with the patient and family members. Guidelines are given with great detail. This rarely is the type of communication that creates the potential for harm to a child. The communication that is wanting is that between the nursing staff and the physicians. Assessments are made, recorded, and even verbally passed on to nurses taking over the responsibility for continued patient care. The failure to include the physicians in abnormal findings or changes in patient assessments can lead to significant adverse outcomes (Wong, 1996).

PEDIATRIC MEDICATION ADMINISTRATION

Medication administration errors accounted for the majority of deaths and injuries in a database research study examining adverse outcomes associated with nursing negligence cases. The majority of pediatric patients experiencing these tragedies were 2 weeks to 3 years of age (Beckmann, 1996).

Faulty technique in parenteral administration of medicine accounted for most injuries, whereas administration of the incorrect dosage or incorrect intravenous solutions accounted for most deaths. The area of concern with unrecognized adverse or toxic effects was secondary only to the liability identified with incorrect dosage (Beckmann, 1996).

The pediatric nurse must be familiar with and competent in using a method of checks and balances in the preparation and administration of medications to children. A commonly used copyrighted form for estimating drug dosages in children is the West Nomogram (West, 1992). When this instrument is not available and medication information is not included with a drug that is unfamiliar to the pediatric nurse, the pharmacist must be called for all pertinent drug reference information. The responsibility for recognizing side effects, adverse reactions, toxicity, and anaphylaxis rests with the nurse administering the drug. (Many current pediatric textbooks have illustrations of the West Nomogram.)

INFORMED CONSENT FOR THE PEDIATRIC PATIENT

In most states, children under 18 years of age are considered to be minors. This designation requires that a parent or legal guardian must be informed concerning treatment needs and that permission must be obtained prior to treatment. The major exception is in life-or-death conditions where the parent or legal guardian is not available to make an immediate decision. In this event, the permission is obtained following the facility's legal guidelines. Oral consent over the telephone can be validated when two witnesses hear the consent given and sign the permission form.

Situations that might arise during hospitalization or treatment that require an additional informed consent declaration include minor or major surgery. When there is an element of risk, such as in diagnostic procedures or medical treatments, a separate consent is required. Other areas that need specifically stated consent include taking photographs and taking the child from the facility against medical advice. The autopsy of a child requires an informed consent except in cases of unexplained death.

The age of pediatric care often extends beyond childhood. In some situations when young adolescents are involved, informed consent can be obtained from the patient. This scenario encompasses the emancipated minor who is legally recognized as having the capacity of an adult. Examples of these persons include the married minor, the unmarried pregnant minor, and the self-supporting minor living away from parental care. Other areas might be recognized by some states on an individual basis. The final example of a minor that does not need parental consent is in the case of child abuse, neglect, or abandonment.

ALLEGATIONS OF PEDIATRIC ABUSE AND NEGLECT

The detection of physical or emotional abuse or neglect in the pediatric patient must be taken seriously and with caution by health care providers. The seriousness is related to early detection and reporting of abuse or neglect to prevent further injury to a child. The caution is directly associated with the high percentage (nearly 50%) of false accusations (Gardner, 1992). Some overreporting can be anticipated due to the general instructions and guidelines that require reporting of suspected cases of abuse or neglect. Because no penalties are applied (usually) for false reporting, reports frequently are made to "hotlines" even when little information, other than the physical signs, is available.

A hotline call might result in the removal of the child from the home setting until an investigation is made by child welfare agency members. This will safeguard a child from continued abuse, but in falsely reported cases, the child might be separated from a caring home environment. Emotional injury to the parents as well as to the child could result from false reporting. Therefore, review of all aspects of the suspected abuse with a trained abuse counselor should be undertaken prior to reporting minor concerns that might prove to be truly accidental injuries. Besharov (1987) found that the social welfare system on child abuse is so overwhelmed with initial calls that many severely abusive situations are not investigated due to time spent in the investigations of non-abuse-related minor accidents that present to emergency departments.

PEDIATRIC PHYSICAL ABUSE

Abuse is the deliberate infliction of physical injury on a child by a caregiver. Whereas this definition is general in scope, child welfare agencies within each state set identification and reporting guidelines.

Three major variables have been identified as precipitating factors to physical abuse of children. The most frequently isolated factors in child physical abuse are (1) characteristics of the parents or caregivers, (2) characteristics of the child, and (3) state of the family environment (Kreitzer, 1981).

Documentation of the physical condition of the child on entering the health care system is essential. Keep the child in a protected environment until a thorough examination and evaluation can be made. Following documentation, the mechanism of reporting the suspected physical abuse is mandated by law. Reporting usually is done through an established local, regional, or statewide hotline system (Potter and Perry, 1995).

PEDIATRIC NEGLECT

Neglect usually is defined as the mistreatment through deprivation of necessities for basic needs and care. Neglect can be physical or emotional (or both) in nature. The physical neglect charge is based on deprivation or omission of necessary care, whereas emotional neglect can be deprivation of essential parental support or even deliberate acts that are devastating to the child's ego. Emotional neglect that is caused by inaction usually involves damage to a child's self-esteem or competence. Garbarino, Guttmann, and Seeley (1986) found that adult conduct consisting of ignoring, isolating, terrorizing, or corrupting a child constitutes emotional neglect. When the social or moral development of a child is misdirected or destroyed, the subversion can lead to a lifetime of antisocial behaviors.

Recording Abuse

Careful recording of objective assessment findings is the best way in which to begin charting the data on a child who is suspected of being abused or neglected. The use of drawings and/or photographs of the physical signs of suspected abuse should accompany the written objective findings. When subjective information is being obtained, it is important to note actual quotes from the child and/or any adult present who is discussing the circumstances surrounding

TABLE 13.1 Documentation in Suspected Child Abuse

History of the incident
1. Day, date, time, and place of the incident
2. Statement of the order of events with times
3. Names of all witnesses and caregivers at the times stated in Item 2
4. Information regarding actions taken during time intervals if treatment was not sought immediately following the event
5. A private interview with the child involved, if possible
6. Private interviews with each adult present at or near the time of the event
7. Observation of the interactions between the child and adults during a group interview; use of quotes from the group interview

Physical assessment findings
1. Location, size, shape, distinguishing colorations or features of marks on the child, use of both written and diagrammatical formats in the record
   Include characteristics of shapes that may match objects such as a belt, a hand, stove burners, a cigarette lighter, and cigarettes
2. Presence of other injuries, old injuries, or other marks on the child's body
3. Tenderness or pain at the area of the injury or in any other areas of the body

the cause for the child's visit. Additional documentation of referral sources, the identity of the exact person receiving the referral, and the immediate outcome of the contact is necessary. Krugman (1989a, 1989b) concluded that any incompatibility between the history and the injury assessed is one of the most important elements in the decision to report a case of suspected abuse. Table 13.1 lists the items that are needed in documenting suspected child abuse.

CONCLUSION

Documentation of nursing care rendered to children and families generally follows the same rules as that rendered to adults. Exceptions are in obtaining informed consent for most medical and diagnostic interventions as well as all surgical interventions. This is similar to the adult pattern of consent but is more specific to signed forms and usually does not include implied consent. Additional exceptions are in cases of emancipated minors.

Medication errors cause most deaths and injuries to pediatric patients, as identified by current litigation studies. Information is available and must be used in safeguarding the pediatric patient from medication mistakes or ignored complications that require action.

Communication with the pediatrician or other health team members is identified as the second most serious cause of litigation for nursing negligence in pediatric damage claims. All pediatric nurses need to identify deficits in nurse-physician communication and initiate quality improvement efforts. Using a continuous quality improvement format in striving for better communication surely will reward all involved in the health care process.

The areas of increasing concern for the pediatric patient center around abuse, neglect, and abandonment. This chapter provided a brief overview of the mechanisms for pediatric nurses to better understand the necessity of the advocacy role. Caution is needed when allegations of abuse are made. The possibility of false allegations can be harmful to the child and family. Agency guidelines that deal with concerns of abuse or neglect are necessary to prevent the damage from inaccurate charges.

This chapter limited the discussion to areas of nursing care that are prominent in litigation literature. By no means was it exhaustive in routine pediatric unit documentation.

CASE STUDY

A 4-month-old girl, Jodie, was brought into the urgent care department of a children's medical center by her mother. The mother reported that the baby had refused to take any formula, juice, or water for the past 18 hours. Over the past several hours, the baby's cry had weakened from a tearful, shrill cry to a tearless, whimpering cry with deep sighs. Jodie's skin was warm to the touch. She exhibited dry mucus membranes with a core temperature of 103.4°F. After Jodie was assessed by the pediatrician, orders were given including one for intravenous (IV) fluids.

The pediatric staff nurse assigned to Jodie proceeded to initiate the venipuncture using a flat Y-shaped tie-down board. The baby's cry intensified and then stopped. When the IV tube was placed, the nurse began to remove the ties and assessed bradypnea. Before the ties were completely removed, Jodie stopped breathing.

The nurse frantically searched the area for an "ambu bag" (forced breathing bag) but failed to identify the pediatric crash box or to call an emergency or "code blue." After failing to locate any resuscitation equipment in the procedure room, she carried the baby to the emergency room in the adjoining hall. Once in the emergency room, Jodie was successfully resuscitated but experienced a profound oxygen deficit. This case was settled out of court for an estimated $2,000,000 for lifelong care due to severe brain damage.

When the depositions were taken, the nurse attending Jodie in the urgent care center indicated she had never completed the required unit orientation to emergency procedures. Although she had been employed for more than 6 months in the urgent care area, she had not sought to complete the orientation packet or classroom discussion on emergency procedures. She felt that the facility was responsible for telling her when she needed to make up this class after she had been absent on the originally scheduled date.

This situation could have been avoided if the nurse had taken personal responsibility for learning vital safety information. The supervisor or manager of the area should have made the class mandatory and not permitted this nurse to have an assignment in which risk of patient safety was present. The facility made changes in new nurse orientation that required completion of all unit skills prior to beginning duty on any patient care unit.

RECORDING PATIENT CARE IN PERIOPERATIVE NURSING

14

Linda L. Zinser-Eagle
Sue E. Meiner

Chapter Outline

Perioperative nursing encompasses three main areas of patient care: preoperative, intraoperative, and postoperative nursing care. Perioperative nursing care begins with the physician's or surgeon's determination that a surgical or other invasive procedure is required. It continues throughout the period of time from that awareness until the patient is considered to have recovered from the surgery or invasive procedure (Association of Operating Room Nurses [AORN], 1998).

The use of the nursing process in perioperative nursing provides the framework for patient care. According to AORN, the patient's medical record should reflect his or her status, nursing diagnoses, interventions, and expected patient outcomes as well as an evaluation of the patient's response to the nursing interventions. As in other nursing specialties, common forms of documentation systems include the use of flow sheets, checklists, and nurses notes. In addition, implant records; laser logs; and surgical sponge, sharp, and instrument count records are commonly used in the perioperative areas (AORN, 1998).

The goal of perioperative nursing is to assist the patient and his or her significant others with attaining a degree of health that is an improvement from the presurgical or preprocedural state of health. This care is given in a variety of settings such as physicians' offices, ambulatory care clinics, and surgical suites within hospitals or freestanding "surgicenters." It is this variety and number of settings through which a patient moves that makes the thoroughness of recording vital to continuity and quality of nursing care and patient outcomes. According to AORN (1998), the perioperative nurse meets the daily challenge to give supportive, efficient, cost-effective nursing care of the highest standards while maintaining documentation of the care.

Although documentation systems differ among perioperative settings, the contents of the pre- and postoperative assessment sheets and the intraoperative record need to be consistent from patient to patient, regardless of the nursing staff member charting. Making each facility's recording reflect the policies and philosophy of the institution and meet the thoroughness of perioperative nursing requires consistent leadership and dissemination of information.

The entire perioperative record, or series of records, should contain the identification of persons providing perioperative patient care. This should include the first initial and surname with title and signature of each person responsible for care. AORN (1998) recommends that perioperative documentation be done by a registered nurse (RN).

LITIGATION FINDINGS
IN PERIOPERATIVE NURSING

Beckmann (1996) identified the most common cause of adverse outcomes within the operating room (OR) as the need for additional surgical intervention. The extra surgeries were related to retained sponges, instruments, or other items that were found to have been closed into body cavities during surgical procedures. The second leading cause of adverse outcomes was performing a procedure on the wrong limb.

PREOPERATIVE PHASE

Establishing a Plan of Care

The patient-centered plan of care is written and provides a guide for nursing actions and the evaluation of goals and outcomes. Preoperative teaching and expected outcomes are to be clearly stated for use by the perioperative team members to provide continuity of care through postoperative teaching. The RN will begin to record the plan of care based on the various patient assessments that include psychosocial, physical, cultural, and learning needs.

Preoperative Assessment

The preoperative assessment may begin in the physician's office when the need for surgery is established. However, depending on the institution, it may be done 1 or 2 days before the procedure at the site of the planned surgery. The perioperative nurse may schedule an interview time with the patient while other preoperative diagnostic tests are being completed. Another method for obtaining the preoperative assessment is by telephone.

An experienced RN, using an appropriate assessment tool, can complete the interview by telephone 1 or 2 days before the scheduled procedure. With the permission of the patient, the nurse may ask for information from family members or significant others if the patient is unable to respond. If the patient is already admitted to the hospital, then the nurse should take the opportunity to see the patient prior to the patient's arrival at the surgical suite.

The preoperative tool also should contain documentation of preoperative instructions given to the patient and the patient's understanding of these instructions. This may include, but is not limited to, any preparation such as special bathing or abstaining from taking any food or fluids by mouth (NPO). It should indicate instructions about medications the patient should hold or take before coming to the facility for surgery.

The nurse also will want to instruct the patient on when and where to arrive if he or she is to arrive on the day of the procedure. If the patient will be discharged home immediately after the procedure, then the patient must be aware that driving after the procedure is unsafe and that arrangements for transportation home are needed.

On the day of the procedure, the plan of care is continued and the patient is reassessed. The time that the patient arrives in the preoperative area should be documented with his or her physical status, psychological status, and general appearance. Notes should include the name of the friend or family member who arrives with the patient, especially if this person is the designated driver to take the patient home. It is useful to note how and where this person can be reached during and after the procedure so that he or she may be given updates on the patient's progress and the results of the surgery. A flow sheet that is not a permanent part of the patient's record may be used to facilitate frequent communication with the patient's significant other or family member and may contain the beeper or phone number at which he or she can be reached.

Orders may be given for preoperative antibiotics, eye drops, or other medications that are given for reasons related to the surgical procedure. Medications and the written or verbal order for them are documented on the preoperative record. Chart 14.1 presents a sample outpatient surgery pre- and postoperative phone call interview form.

Consent Forms

Documentation of the presence of the consent form for surgery is vital. This means that the responsibility of obtaining the informed consent resides with the physician who is doing the procedure. Informed consent means that the patient has received a thorough explanation and understands the risks, the alternative methods of treatment, and the probability of successful outcome of the procedure. The nurse cannot obtain the consent; the nurse can only witness the patient's signature on the form. More than one consent might be required for a procedure. For example, the patient might have to sign separate consents for sterilization, to receive blood products, for experimental techniques, and/or for radiation therapy, depending on the policies of the institution.

Nurses verify that the consent correctly indicates the procedure about to be done (e.g., consent should clearly indicate left or right breast biopsy). The nurse should verify this information verbally with the patient. Chapter 10 provided additional elements of informed consent.

Relevant Past Medical and Surgical History

The physician's diagnosis and indication of informed consent and intent to do the specific procedure must be included as required by state and institutional requirements. These often are faxed to the place of the surgical procedure and are copied onto plain paper if the fax machine uses heat-sensitive paper. A clear copy is needed for the permanent record.

The importance of recording the past medical and surgical history of the patient cannot be overlooked. Areas that need to be recorded are past surgical interventions, preexisting medical problems, laboratory results, medication history, physical assessment, allergies to drugs or food, and latex sensitivity. Other specific questions might need to be answered concerning the nature of the procedure being done.

A documentation system that allows one form to be used by anesthesia, physicians/surgeons, and nursing is quite useful to avoid duplication of questions. When multiple professionals ask the same items, patients and family members tend to have increased stress in thinking that members of the surgical team are not talking to each other.

Perioperative Assessment

Components of the perioperative assessment incorporate physical and psychological assessments, medical data, diagnostic reports, nursing care data, and discharge information for follow-up care. Each of these areas has several items for assessment that will lead to establishing a plan of care and nursing diagnoses appropriate to the needs of the patient.

Physiological Assessment

Besides the physician's physical examination, the perioperative nurse will perform a physical assessment of the patient. Physical assessment can be made using the body systems medical model or the functional nursing model. Among the parameters suggested by Atkinson and Fortunato (1996) are the following physiological areas:

1. Allergies, vital signs, and sensory impairments
2. Nutritional and metabolic status, weight, and height
3. Mobility, range of motion, and prosthetics (internal or external)
4. Elimination patterns (bowel and bladder)
5. Skin condition
6. Sleep, rest, and exercise patterns
7. Medications/drugs (prescribed, over-the-counter, illegal, and alcohol)

Chart 14.2 provides a sample preoperative assessment/plan form.

Psychological Assessment

A psychological assessment is aimed toward the patient's general perceptions about surgery, coping and defense mechanisms, support systems in place, attention and concentration, reasoning, attitude, and motivation. The importance of this assessment is in direct association with the psychological crisis that can exist for the surgical patient. Surgery often is associated with anxiety attacks, feelings of powerlessness, and even despair (Kneedler and Dodge, 1991).

Identification of ineffective coping skills that may lead to pathological anxiety during the perioperative period might require crisis intervention referral and a specific plan of care to address this problem (Aguilera, 1997). Seeking a spiritual adviser referral should be documented on the perioperative assessment and care form.

CHART 14.1. Sample Outpatient Surgery Preoperative and Postoperative Phone Call Interview Form

---

PRE-OP PHONE CALL INTERVIEW

DATE OF CALL: ___/___/___ Time/Initials: 1ˢᵗ ____/___; 2ⁿᵈ ___/___ ‖ __ no phone #; __ incorrect #; __ line
Busy X ___; ___ No answer X ____ ‖ __ Pt. returned call;
Answering machine - asked to return call/basic instructions given (circle)
Patient Name:_____ Age:___ Sex:___ Phone #: Home: _____ Work #: _____
Surgery date: ___/___/___; Time: ____ Arrival @ ____; per MD ___. Surgeon: _____
Procedure: _____
anesthesia: ___ general; ___ epidural; ___ spinal; ___ regional; MAC ___; A/C ___; IV sedation: ___; Local: ___.
Status: ___ OP; ___ ADM.
Have you had any testing done in the past month / in preparation for your procedure? __ yes; __ no; __ N/A;
Labs: _____; EKG / CXR (circle) in past 6 months? __ yes; __ no; __ N/A.
Primary Care Physician / Internist: _____ph #: _____
TESTING NEEDED: _____
__ Basic Pre-OP instructions given   (recommend no smoking before surgery)
            Location of entrance and admission desk; Bring insurance cards/forms: __; workers' comp. __
            Wear clean, loose, comfortable clothing (consider bandages); Following shower or bath DO NOT
            apply lotions or cosmetics, DO NOT wear or bring jewelry or valuables, DO bring case for glasses
            or contacts
            __ N/A crutches - past training / needs training / bring (circle)
            __ N/A NPO - after Midnight or 8 hrs prior to surgery
            __ N/A Someone available to drive pt. home;
            no driving X 24 hrs - __ yes; __ no.
            __ N/A someone available to stay w/pt. @ home p surgery
            estimated length of procedure, recovery, D/C / RM (circle)
            __ address advanced directives: pt. has one __ yes; __ no.
            will bring in a copy? ___ yes; __ no; __ N/A.
            Would like: to make one/info. only (circle)
            upon adm.__ yes; __ no; __ N/A.
            Admitting / Pastoral Care notified: _ yes; _ no; __ N/A.
            __ pt. / significant other verbalizes understanding of instructions
Pre-op evaluation for nursing and anesthesia initiated:___; Discharge progress form initiated: __;
Special instructions:_____
_____
_____
__ take the following meds in a.m. w/sip of H2O: _____
_____
_____
_Comments:_____
_____
_____
_____

                                    Signature of the RN interviewer

---

Other Areas of Preoperative Preparation

    Confirmation of the examination by the physician and the anesthesia provider
should be recorded. Diagnostic tests and laboratory results ordered as preoperative

CHART 14.1 *Continued*

POST-OP PHONE CALL INTERVIEW: Patient's Name: _____ I.D. # _____
This form must be attached to the OUTPATIENT SURGERY DEPARTMENT PRE-OP PHONE INTERVIEW

Date: _/_/_; Time: _____

Felling well: __; __ back to work/school
tired __; fatigued: __; N/V: __
Comments: _____
_____
_____

Pain - none: __; relieved by RX: __ ;
relieved by OTC med. ___;
pain, uncomfortable: ___.
Comments: _____
_____
_____

Nausea, Vomiting. - none: __;
Relieved by RX: ___;
tolerating liquids: ___; Dr. aware: ___;
Comments:_____
_____
_____

Dressing, none: ___; Drainage:_____;
Dr. aware:___; Dry & Intact: _____;
Comments:_____
_____
_____

Incision covered: __ yes; __ no; __ none
no drainage: __; red & swollen: __
drainage: ___; suture/staples intact: __;
Comments: _____
_____

Temperature normal: __; temp.>100: __
Comments: _____
_____
_____

Dr.'s appt. made: _____;
instructed to call for post-op appt.: ___;
Special instructions: _____
_____
_____

Verbalized understanding of instructions:
___ yes; ___ no; Comments: _____
_____
_____

Referred to: ___ anesthesia; ___ MD.
Anesthesia notified: ___ yes; ___ no.
Who: _____

time: _____ on __/__/__
Nurses Notes:
Comments:
_____
_____
_____
_____
_____
_____
_____
_____
_____
_____

signature of the RN interviewer

---

tests should be available and recorded. Drug allergies and latex sensitivity should be boldly noted on the record, and an identification armband should be placed on the patient. This may vary according to specific institutional policies.

Transportation from the preparation area should be documented as to the method used and the time the patient departs. All of this is most easily accomplished with a checklist that should follow the patient through the perioperative process.

CHART 14.2 Sample Preoperative Assessment/Plan Form

PATIENT'S STAMP HERE

Physical Assessment: (only check marks indicate a deficit, no check marks indicate no deficit or not applicable to patient)

DATE: _____; TIME: _____

Vital signs: T. ___; P. ___; R. __; BP. __/__;   O2 sat. ___%; Ht. ___; Wt. ___; NPO since: _____
IV fluids: device used:_____; fluid: _____; site: _____; time of insertion: _____; who: _____
Cardiovascular: __ abn. blood; __ abn. ECG; __ s/p MI; __ s/p open heart surg.; other: _____
Respiratory: __ abn. X-ray; __ History of resp. compromise - explain: _____
Consciousness: __ sedated;   __ restless; __crying; __ confused; __ agitated; __ combative.
Elimination: __ foley;   __ incontinent; __ abn. UA; other: _____
Mobility: __ paralysis; __ arthritis; __ obesity; __ traction present; other: _____
Communication - Sensory: __ language; __ hearing; __ aphasic; __ mute;   __ vision; __ pain;
        other: _____
Skin: *(Use diagrams below according to the code at the left of the figures)*
Prosthesis or Implants: __ glasses; __ dentures; __ contact lenses; __ hearing aid(s)- L:__/R:__; __ pacemaker;
        ortho: ___ and describe: _____

Psychological: Coping - __ accepting; __ withdrawn; __ talkative; other: _____
Comfort: ___ Position; __ temperature; __ Noise; __;   other: _____

PLACE A CHECK MARK ON THE ITEMS THAT ARE APPLICABLE:
Verification Noted: __ I.D. present; __ bracelet; __ chart; __ Chart complete; ___ consent form signed with witness.
Pre-operative orders checked: ___ yes; who checked: _____; signature: _____time: _____

SKIN ASSESSMENT/NURSING INTERVENTION

Potential Nursing Diagnosis:
Impaired Skin Integrity
Indicate appropriate code on
the anatomical diagram

A -Abrasion
BL -Blister
BR -Bruise
B -Burn
C -Contusion
D -Decubitus
E -Erythema
G -Graft
H -Hematoma
L -Laceration
PA -Papule
PU -Pustule
R -Rash
S -Scar
Comments:

Nursing Diagnosis	*Outcomes expected*	*Intervention*	*Evaluation*
1. Anxiety	Ventilate feelings	OR protocol explained Patients questions addressed	Verbalizes understanding
2. Potential alteration of body temperature	Body temperature maintained	Area of exposure limited Warm blanket provided	Temperature remains within normal limits

INTRAOPERATIVE PHASE

The intraoperative phase of patient care usually is recorded on what is called the OP record. The intraoperative nurse ideally is aware of the preoperative assessment prior to the patient's arrival in the surgery area. The intraoperative nurse might meet the patient for the first time in an area outside the surgical suite called the holding area. But even prior to this meeting, the intraoperative nurse will have begun to form a plan of care based on the individual needs of the patient and the technical needs of performing the specific procedure. Chart 14.3 illustrates a sample OP record. Ideally, the record contains a method for documenting assessment, diagnosis, implementation, and evaluation of care.

Basic Elements of Operating Room Charting

The essentials of any OP record begin with checking the patient's name and identification for accuracy. This is followed by entering the complete date, time of entering the OR suite, preoperative diagnosis, and surgical procedure to be performed. Persons on the surgical team are listed by name and title such as the anesthesia provider, scrub person, and circulating RN.

Descriptions of the patient's overall skin condition on arrival at and at discharge from the perioperative suites is essential. Any scars, rashes, bruising, or other skin conditions must be recorded. This is the first important step in assessing, planning, and implementing the positioning of the patient. A patient with poor skin quality might have to have parts of the OR table padded more than usual. This is important to note in the positioning section of the record. Document that the physician is told about any special skin observations that might require the changing of the incision site or affect the use of equipment or positioning devices (Atkinson and Fortunato, 1996; Fogg, 1993). (See the skin assessment component of Chart 14.1.)

Safe patient positioning requires knowledge and teamwork. The position must be physiologically safe for the patient while permitting the surgeon optimal exposure for the procedure. Individual patient limitations must be considered in planning for the procedure. Adequate equipment, personnel, and teamwork are required for patient safety in positioning. Recording the basic position and repositioning of the patient, positioning devices used, location and restraint of extremities, safety belts used and location, and padding is essential. The use of a checklist or flow sheet that requires responding to items listed for the specific purpose of monitoring the safety of positioning is highly recommended.

Recording the application and placement of the safety belt is essential. Restraint use protocols are exempt in the OR. However, the usual institutional rules are in effect in the preoperative holding areas and postoperative care areas.

The presence and/or disposition of sensory aids such as hearing aids, glasses, and contact lenses, or the presence of other prostheses, must be recorded. If the patient is awake and the devices do not interfere with the access to the surgical site, then these devices may remain in place during the procedure. The surgeon and the anesthesia professional have the final say in whether to retain sensory aids or other prostheses during surgery. Chart 14.4 provides an example of an intraoperative nursing care plan.

CHART 14.3 Sample Intraoperative (OP) Record

PATIENT'S STAMP HERE

DATE: _____; TIME: _____
Review of Pre-Operative Assessment and Plan form completed: ___ yes;
Signature & credentials of reviewer: _____
Comments: _____
_____

Allergies: __ yes; __ no. If yes, list: _____
Verification Noted: __ I.D. present; __ bracelet; __ chart; __ Chart complete; ___ consent form signed with witness.
Pre-operative orders checked: ___ yes; who checked: _____; signature: _____time: _____
Name and credentials of accompanying party during patient transfer to the OR: _____

*NURSING DIAGNOSIS: potential for anxiety r/t knowledge deficit; GOAL: demonstrates decreased anxiety;
PLAN/INTERVENTION: provide clear explanations; provide caring and supportive attitude; communicate patient
concerns to health care team members; remain with patient during induction; EVALUATION: demonstrates an
understanding of explanations and instructions.*

		PT IN OR		PT OUT		☐ X-RAY _____ ☐ NA LASER _____ ☐ NA			
PROCEDURE START	1.	PROCEDURE STOP	1.	PROCEDURE START	2	PROCEDURE STOP 2	POST-OP DIAGNOSIS		
PRE-OP DIAGNOSIS							ANESTHETIC ROUTE	☐ GEN ET ☐ GEN MASK ☐ MAC ☐ LOC ☐ SPINAL/EPID ☐ REGIONAL ☐ BLOCK TYPE _____ ☐ NONE	
PROCEDURE							SCRUB NURSES/TITLE/INITIAL ☐ NA	TIME IN/OUT	TIME IN/OUT	TIME IN/OUT
	PRIMARY PROCEDURE		SECONDARY PROCEDURE							
SURGEON										
1ST ASSISTANT										
OTHER										
ATTENDING ANESTHESIOLOGIST		RELIEF					CIRCULATING NURSES/TITLE/INITIAL			
RESIDENT ANESTHESIOLOGIST		RELIEF								
ANESTHETIST		RELIEF								
OBSERVERS ☐ NA										

NURSES NOTES:_____
_____
_____
_____
_____
_____signature & credentials: _____

Nursing Diagnosis	*Outcomes expected*	*Intervention*	*Evaluation*
1. Potential for injury	Patient will be injury free	Safety restraint	No injuries
2. Potential for infection	Infection free	Sterile technique	No breaks in sterile technique

---

Skin Preparation

Documentation in the OP record should include the condition of the skin
around the surgical site, any hair removal, the name or type of skin preparation

CHART 14.4 Intraoperative Assessment/Plan/Implementation/Evaluation With Nursing Diagnosis

INTRA-OP ASSESSMENT/PLAN	IMPLEMENTATION	EVALUATION
Thermal/Cooling Blanket Body Temp. Altered, Potential ☐ None	Serial #:_____Temp. Setting _____ Setting ordered by:_____	Y N ☐ ☐ Temp. WNL ☐ ☐ Site Clear
Position/Devices Injury, Potential (Positioning)	☐ Supine L ARMS R ☐ Safety belt ☐ Lami talbe ☐ Sandbag ☐ Prone ☐ at side ☐ ☐ Pillows ☐ Chest rolls ☐ Foam wedge ☐ Lithotomy ☐ ext <90° ☐ ☐ Vac pac ☐ Ax. roll ☐ Tape ☐ Jackknife ☐ arm bds ☐ ☐ Cane stirrups ☐ Egg crate ☐ Shoulder roll ☐ Rt. Lat'l ☐ other ☐ ☐ Blankets ☐ Hand table ☐ Peg board ☐ Lt. Lat'l ☐ Fx table ☐ Donut ☐ Allen stirrups ☐ Other ☐ Kidney table ☐ Headrest Comments: ☐ Arthroscopic leg holder	
IV (local cases only) Fluid Volume Deficit, Potential ☐ None/NA ☐ See Anesthesia	☐ Inserted in Ambulatory Surgery—see Pre-Operative Assessment/Plan ☐ Inserted in OR: Catheter size:_____ Site:_____ Fluid: _____ Inserted by:_____	_____ cc infused Y N ☐ ☐ Patent ☐ ☐ Site clear ☐ ☐ DC'd in OR
EKG (local cases only) Cardiac Output, Potential Decrease ☐ None/NA	☐ EKG monitored during surgery	Y N ☐ ☐ Sinus Rhythm ☐ ☐ Pads removed
ESU Injury, Potential (Burn) ☐ None	☐ Monopolar generator #_____ Ground pad site: ☐ Rt ☐ Lt Coag:_____ Cut:_____ Anterior ☐ Posterior ☐ ☐ Bipolar generator #_____ Arm ☐ Shoulder ☐ Setting:_____ Leg ☐ Buttocks ☐ Skin Condition Preop:_____ Ground Pad Type:_____	Y N ☐ ☐ Pad site clear
Tourniquet Injury, Potential (Skin/Perfusion) ☐ None	Rt Lt ☐ Arm ☐ Leg Up @_____ Applied by:_____ Down @_____ Setting:_____ Number:_____	Y N ☐ ☐ Circulation intact ☐ ☐ Site clear
Hair Removal Infection, Potential Injury, Potential ☐ None	☐ Shaved by:_____ Septisol ☐ Betadine ☐ Other ☐ _____ ☐ Clipped by:_____	Y N ☐ ☐ Site clear
Skin Prep Infection, Potential ☐ None	☐ Iodophor scrub ☐ Betadine gel ☐ Hibiclens ☐ Vag Prep ☐ Iodophor solution ☐ Alcohol ☐ Phisohex ☐ Other ☐ Duraprep ☐ Iodine/Alcohol ☐ Septisol Prepped by:_____	Y N ☐ ☐ Reaction ☐ ☐ Asepsis maintained
Vessel Cross Clamp Perfusion Deficit, Potential ☐ None/NA	☐ Vessel:_____ On:_____ Off:_____ On:_____ Off:_____ ☐ Cardiopulmonary Bypass On:_____ Off:_____ On:_____ Off:_____ Perfusionist:_____	Y N ☐ ☐ Circulation Intact
Circulatory Support Devices Perfusion Deficit. Potential ☐ None/NA	☐ Sequential Compression Device #_____ ☐ TEDs: ☐ Thigh ☐ Knee ☐ Other	Y N ☐ ☐ Circulation Intact
Catheters Urinary Elimination, Alteration ☐ None	☐ Insitu Type:_____ Size:_____ ☐ Urethral ☐ Suprapubic Inserted by:_____ Character of Urine:_____	Y N ☐ ☐ In w/o diff. Output:_____cc ☐ See anes rec ☐ Removed in OR
Dressing Skin Integrity Alteration ☐ None	☐ Telfa ☐ Sponges ☐ Dermaform tape ☐ Splint ☐ Other ☐ Adaptic ☐ Fluffs ☐ Cloth tape ☐ Cast ☐ Xeroform ☐ Kerlex/Kling ☐ Paper tape ☐ Immobilizer ☐ Steri-strips ☐ Ace/Coban ☐ Elastoplast ☐ Fox shield ☐ Primapore/coverlet ☐ Bandaids ☐ Peri-pad ☐ Eye patch	Y N ☐ ☐ Dressing dry and intact

Discharge to: ☐ PACU ☐ ASD ☐ ICU ☐ Floor Room #_____ ☐ _____

Transported via: ☐ Stretcher ☐ Bed ☐ Crib ☐ Wheelchair ☐ Ambulatory ☐ Eye Cart ☐ Wagon ☐_____

Oxygen on discharge: ☐ None/NA ☐ Running at _____L/min via ☐ Cannula ☐ Mask ☐ ET Signature:_____RN

solution used, the area prepared for incision, skin reaction (positive or negative), and the name of the person "prepping" the skin.

Electrosurgical Units

The most frequently used piece of electrical equipment in the OR is the electrosurgical unit (ESU). Electrosurgery uses an active electrode that delivers high-frequency electrical energy that cuts and/or provides hemostasis. Depending on the type of current used, a disposable dispersive electrode or grounding pad is placed on the patient's body to safely return current to the machine. It is vital to specifically document the location of the placement of the grounding pad. Some institutions also document the name of the person who places this pad. It is necessary to document the identification number of the ESU and the range of the power settings used during the procedure. Assessment of the condition of the skin at the grounding pad site before and after the use of ESU is recommended.

Sequential Compression Equipment

Sequential pneumatic compression (SPC) devices frequently are used during surgery when the patient is at risk for deep vein clotting. Areas to be recorded in the OP record are the type of device, the specific unit number of the device used, time started, pressure and cycle settings, and time stopped. The patient's skin circulatory response to the SPC must be present following the discontinuance of the device. (The unit probably will be discontinued in the postanesthesia care unit (PACU) or in the patient's room several days after surgery.)

Body Temperature Protection

Body heat is lost during the preoperative period. In most hospitals' surgical units, monitoring the patient's thermoregulation throughout the intraoperative phase is the responsibility of the anesthesia provider. The RN is responsible for recording the use of temperature-regulating devices such as the "bear huggers" used by the anesthesia provider to warm the patient.

Recording the Use of Lasers

The word *laser* is an acronym for *l*ight *a*mplification by *s*timulated *e*mission of *r*adiation. Lasers can be hazardous. Therefore, the safety and recording issues surrounding the use of lasers in surgery require special mention. Recording the use of the laser may occur on the interoperative form or on a separate laser log form that is attached to the OR record. A copy of this form must be maintained as a permanent laser log in the OR suite.

Documentation of laser care requires the listing of the patient's name, date, time, surgeon, procedure, type of laser used, length of use, and wattage. The

CHART 14.5 Sample Laser Safety Log Form

	PATIENT'S STAMP HERE

Date: _____; Time: _____.

Surgeon: _____.

Assistants: _____; Scrub: _____

Circulator: _____; Preoperative Diagnosis: _____

Procedure: _____

LASER DELIVERY MODE:

___ MICRO MANIPULATOR;   ___ LAPAROSCOPE;   LENS: _____
___ FREE HAND;   ____ PROBE;   FIBER SIZE: _____
___ ENDOSCOPE   TYPE: _____

PATIENT SAFETY PRECAUTIONS:

Eye Protection: ___ Goggles;   ___ Moist towels;   ___ Moist eye pads;   ___ Tape;
                         ___ Water soluble ointment.
Prep Solution dried: ___ Yes;   ___ No;   ___ N/A
Draping of incision: ___ Disposable;   ___Wet Linen;   ___ Combination drape.
Saline water in room: ___ Yes.
Moist sponges: ___ Used on surgical field;   ___ Not used;   ___ in rectum;   ___ in throat.

PERSONNEL SAFETY PRECAUTIONS:

___ Signage posted on all entrance doors to operating room.
___ Protective eye wear worn by all persons in the operating room; or if not: ___ no;   ___ N/A
___ Eye safety filter: ___ yes;   ___ no; or ___ N/A
___ Smoke evacuation method on during laser usage.
___ If applicable, type of window covering used, name: _____

Signature of person completing this laser-use check-list: _____title: _____
Signature of person testing the Laser: _____title: _____

TIME	WATTS	MODE	TIME	WATTS	MODE

times of beginning and ending of use, names of persons using the laser, type of laser, length of total use, and wattage also need to be recorded (Atkinson and Fortunato, 1996). Chart 14.5 illustrates a sample laser safety log form.

Recording the Placement of a Tourniquet

When a tourniquet is needed during a surgical procedure, the type, time of placement, location on the patient, padding used, pressure setting, name of person who placed the tourniquet, and name of person responsible for monitoring the patient's condition are recorded in the OP record. When the tourniquet is removed, the time and patient's condition must be entered to complete the record.

Sponge, Sharp, and Instrument Counts

Of paramount importance in the OR is the accuracy of counting all sponges, instruments, and needles used during a surgical case procedure. Inadvertently leaving one of these items inside a patient is a life-threatening and costly mistake. The best means of preventing this occurrence is to properly perform a count of sponges, needles, blades, instruments, and miscellaneous items at several key points during surgery. This must be completely documented.

AORN recommends that initial counts be taken before a procedure to provide baseline data. Any additional sponges, needles, or instruments added to the surgical field are immediately recorded as added items. Usually, two additional counts are done as the surgeon is ready to close the deep cavity and during skin closure or at the end of surgery. Another recommended time for completing a count is when a permanent relief scrub or circulating RN takes over during a continuing procedure. The names of the relief scrub and circulating nurse performing the counts, as well as the status of the counts (e.g., correct), must be recorded clearly for each count done during the procedure.

In case of an incorrect count, a thorough search of the surgical field and room is done. The surgeon is notified if the count remains unresolved, and all actions taken must be recorded. If necessary, an X-ray may be taken to find the missing item in the patient. The results of the X-ray are recorded on the OR record, the count is recorded as unresolved, and the names of the relief scrub and circulating RN are recorded. If a count cannot be done due to an emergent situation, then this is to be recorded on the OP record. Chart 14.6 provides a sample operative data form.

Medications Administered During Surgery

Any medication given to the surgeon to administer to the patient at the surgical site are documented on the OP record as to name, dosage, time, and route. These medications are checked prior to administration by the circulating RN and the scrub nurse. In the case of medication used by the surgeon for regional anesthesia (e.g., Lidocaine, Marcaine), the surgeon also should check

CHART 14.6 Sample Operative Data Form

	Patient's Stamp Here

Name: _____; **Date:** _____; **OR room:** _____;
Medical Record #: _____; Major: ___; Minor: ___.
Category: ___ Elective; ___ Emergency; ___ Add-on; ___ Cancel.
Surgeon(s): _____
Scrub Personnel: 1st: ___   . _____; 2nd _____
        3rd. _____;Relief Scrub: 1st. _____; 2nd. _____
Circulating Nurse(s): _____
Relief/Time: _____
Anesthesia Adm. by: _____ supervised by: _____
Other personnel (students, etc.):_____
Anesthesia: ___ none; ___ parabulbar; ___ general; ___ cervical block; ___ caudal; ___ spinal;
        ___ epidural; ___ regional; ___ IV sedation; ___ local; ___ MAC.
Times: In room: _____; Incision: _____; Wound closure: _____

Pre-op Diagnosis:

Procedure:

Post-op Diagnosis:

	Yes x	No	Drains:		Packing:	Laser:
Specimens:	▢	▢	▢ None	▢ J-Vac	▢ None	Type:_____
Frozen Section	▢	▢	▢ Salem Sump	▢ Jackson-Pratt	▢ Iodoform	Setting/
Culture	▢	▢	▢ Penrose	▢ T-Tube	▢ Plain	Watts:: _____
Location:			▢ Hemovac	▢ Chest Tube	▢ Other:	Safety
			▢ Abramson	▢ Clear Drain	Location of Pack:	Precautions: ▢Yes ▢No
			▢ Solcotrans	▢ ICP		Serial #:_____
			▢ Stryker	▢ Other		Time-Begin: End:

Count Items: ▢ None	Sponge Counts		Sharps Counts		Instrument Counts
	Initial		Initial		Initial
	1st		1st		1st
	Final		Final		Final

If incorrect: ▢ X-ray taken If no, explain:

Medications/Irrigations ▢ None				Vital Signs (local)				
Drug/Type	Dose/Amount ROA/Site Admin by Time			Time	B/P	P	R	O2 sat

Implants: ▢ None ▢ Labels on back   Special Equipment Used: X-ray ▢ C-arm ▢
Type:

the container for name, dosage, and other properties that are essential to some classifications of medications prior to delivering the medication to the field.

The use of conscious sedation/analgesia is not covered in this chapter. Chapter 10 provided information on conscious sedation given in the emergency department. AORN (1998) established guidelines for RNs managing patients receiving conscious sedation/analgesia. When these guidelines are followed, safe, effective, quality patient care can be maintained.

Handling and Recording Specimens and Cultures

Some institutions use a separate form to record patient specimens and cultures taken during a surgical procedure. Notation that a specimen was obtained and where it was sent should be recorded on the intraoperative record. After surgery, this may be attached to a separate log book that contains the record of specimens. It is double-checked for disposition when specimens are removed to pathology.

The discussion of specimens that have special disposition is not included in this chapter. Those specimens include items not routinely sent to pathology, such as those disposed of in the OR, and specimens sent to research laboratories with the patient's consent. Specimens for legal evidence or police investigation was briefly discussed in Chapter 10.

Recording Implants

Implants and orthopedic prostheses may be recorded on separate forms that are attached to the intraoperative record. A copy of the form is maintained in the OR to track the specific implant. Each item used must be recorded as a separate implant. The form records the exact item, manufacturer, lot number, serial number, size, and location of the implant. An example is the implantation of a joint into the patient. The joint may have several components, each of which is recorded separately on the form.

Recording Additional Personnel in the Operating Room

Special equipment such as X-ray or fluoroscopy may be used for specific procedures. The first initial, surname, and title of the person operating the machine are recorded on the OP record. Any other professional or nonprofessional personnel (e.g., students, guests, equipment representatives) need to be recorded on the OP record.

Recording Wound Classifications

At the end of the procedure, the nurse will document the classification of the surgical wound on the OP record. The usual four types of wound classifications are clean, clean contaminated, contaminated, or dirty/infected. The exact definitions of these terms can be found in the Glossary.

TABLE 14.1 Items That Must Be Double-Checked in Blood Administration

1. Patient's name and identification number
2. Assigned surgical unit/hospital number
3. Unit of blood or blood product number
4. Date of blood collection
5. Date of cross-matching

Anesthesia Classification Documentation

AORN (1998) recommends that the classification of anesthesia be included on the OP record. This information is easily documented by checking a box on a preprinted form. (See Chart 14.3 for this component on the sample form.)

Recording Drains or Tubes

The nurse should document the types, sizes, and locations of any tubes or drains placed during surgery. The types, colors, and amounts of drainage from these tubes also should be recorded.

Recording Administration of Blood or Blood Products

Loss of blood and body fluids accompanies any surgical procedure. Recording the estimated blood loss is important for replacement fluids to be calculated. The surgeon and/or anesthesiologist are responsible for this estimate. In some OP records, the nurse records the estimated loss that is verbally given at the end of the procedure.

When blood or blood products are used during or after an elective surgery, a laboratory test called *cross-matching* must be in the facility's blood bank. An exception is superficial surgery in which blood loss is expected to be insignificant.

Surgical facilities have a required protocol for verifying that the blood has been checked against the cross-matched specimen and is correctly labeled. The perioperative nurse is responsible for double-checking the blood or blood products for accuracy along with the person administering the blood (usually the anesthesia provider). Table 14.1 lists items to be checked with blood or blood products. Documentation of the transfusion is done according to the institution's policies and may be accomplished on a separate form.

Alternatives to Donor Blood Transfusion

The technique known as autotransfusion is used in many surgical services. The patient's own blood is obtained during the procedure. The blood is pro-

cessed and returned to the patient. Another alternative to donor blood transfusions is autologous transfusion. The patient donates blood prior to the scheduled
surgery. It is retained for use during or after the operation. The transfusion record
will identify blood that is autotransfusion or autologous in origin. Special
protocols and documentation are used by many facilities with outside contracts
to cell saver companies.

Nurses Notes

The intraoperative record should have an area for recording any unusual
occurrences pertinent to perioperative patient outcomes. If a checklist is not on
the form, then the notes need to be written in the nurses notes area. The
perioperative record should include the time that the surgery was finished, the
method of transporting from the procedural room, the destination, and the staff
member who accompanied the patient from the area.

POSTOPERATIVE PHASE

After the procedure is completed, the patient is transferred to a PACU. The plan
of care established in the preoperative phase will provide information related to
special equipment needs, potential complications associated with the surgical
procedure, and unique patient considerations. These data will provide the PACU
nurse with a continuation of the plan of care specific to recovery from anesthesia.
Included in, but not limited to, this record will be a scale for recording the
patient's level of alertness, breathing, ability to move and other criteria of
recovery, level of pain, and any nausea or vomiting. This record also should
contain documentation of a physician's discharge order from the PACU. Chart
14.7 illustrates patient monitoring in the PACU.

OUTPATIENT SURGERY INSTRUCTIONS

In the outpatient setting, the nurse must record patient and/or family teaching
that includes postoperative orders, information on signs and symptoms of
problems and complications, and instructions for emergent care. Other instructions need to include the types or limitations of activities, information regarding
seeing the physician in the office or clinic for follow-up care, and care of the
wound site (if applicable). Time is needed to instruct on resuming or beginning
medications and on essential medication information related to any new prescriptions.

CHART 14.7 Postanesthesia Care Unit (PACU) Record Form

PATIENT'S STAMP HERE

Date: _____

| TIME |
| TEMP |
| O₂ SAT |
| EKG |

Vital signs graph (TEMP △, RESP ○, PULSE ●, SYSTOLIC ∨, DIASTOLIC ∧) scale 0–220

TREATMENT	TIME START	TIME DISC	NURSE INIT
O₂			

AIRWAY TYPE

ANESTHESIA REPORT RECEIVED & REVIEWED ☐

OPERATIVE PROCEDURE

INTRAOPERATIVE COMPLICATIONS

PMH

ALLERGIES

TYPE	OUTPUT	TOTAL OUTPUT	FLUID DEFECIT	AGE	WT.

LOCATION	INTAKE	TOTAL INTKAE

MEDICATIONS

TIME	DRUG	DOSE	ROUTE	NURSE INIT

NURSE'S NOTES

TIME		TIME	

POST ANESTHESIA RECOVERY SCORE

ASSESS	ADMISSION	HOURLY	DISCHARGE
TIME			
ACTIVITY			
RESPIRATION			
CIRCULATION			
CONSCIOUSNESS			
COLOR			
TOTAL			

COMFORT SCORE / **EMESIS SCORE**

Crying= | Score≥1 _____
Agitation | Complications
Pain complaints
Score≥3 _____

ANESTHESIA RELEASE NOTES

Transfer to: _____ Condition: _____ PACU Nurse's Signature

The patient's understanding of instructions, or the understanding of significant others who are present during the instructions, is required prior to discharge. The signature of the patient or responsible person receiving the instructions needs to be placed on the instruction sheets, with a copy retained by the facility.

Other areas that need to be noted include the patient's ability to eat or drink; presence of nausea; ability to void (urinate); and means, time, and person responsible for transportation from the recovery area. Chart 14.8 illustrates a sample outpatient discharge instruction form.

AORN (1998) recommends that policies regarding documentation in the perioperative setting be reviewed and revised as needed on at least an annual basis. This is best done by a committee made up of members of the perioperative team.

CONCLUSION

Perioperative nursing includes the preoperative, intraoperative, and postoperative phases of patient care surrounding surgery. Nursing care given throughout these phases of care is guided by the nursing process. The perioperative nurse provides patient advocacy during periods when the surgical person is unable to perform self-protective measures. The handling of surgical instruments is a minimal component of this complex specialty. Recording in the medical record before, during, and after a surgical experience is detail oriented and comprises a vast amount of critical thinking skills.

The perioperative nurse's activities reflect the psychological, social, and physiological nursing care that is the direct result of surgical interventions. The presentation of perioperative nursing in this chapter represented those elements noted in various legal claims originating from perioperative nursing. The extent of logs, forms, checklists, flow sheets, and narrative forms used throughout the perioperative phases cannot be presented in a brief manner.

CASE STUDY

Mr. N, a 45-year-old man, was admitted for an elective cholecystectomy (gallbladder removal). His weight was 285 pounds, and his height was 5 feet 7 inches. He had recovered from four gallbladder attacks over a period of 2 years and elected to have the cholecystectomy to prevent an emergency procedure in the future.

The procedure had required more than three times the usual amount of absorbent sponges due to a large amount of blood and body fluids lost during the early part of the procedure. Prior to the first cavity closure (second count), the circulating nurse was unsure of the count by one absorbent sponge. The surgeon wanted to proceed to the next level of closure, attributing the unresolved count to the large quantity of saturated sponges in

CHART 14.8 Outpatient Discharge Instructions

Date: _____ ; Time: _____ .

Anesthesia type: __ general / sedation;   or __ local.

Via: __ ambulatory;   __ wheelchair;   __ stretcher.

PATIENT'S STAMP HERE

DISCHARGE INSTRUCTIONS:

___ DO NOT drive, operate machinery, or consume alcohol for the next 24 hours.
___ DO NOT make any legal decisions for the next 24 hours.
___ DO NOT smoke for the next 24 hours unless in the presence of someone else.
___ Stay with a responsible person tonight.

ACTIVITY: ___ NO RESTRICTIONS;   ___ LIGHT ACTIVITY;   ___ KEEP _____ EXTREMITY ELEVATED;
___ USE CRUTCHES;   ___ USE SLING;   Other: _____

MEDICATIONS: ___ Continue Present medications;   ___ New Prescriptions given to patient;   ___ none required;
___ Discharge medications as ordered;   ___ Take usual medications for discomfort;
___ Other: _____
_____

DIET: ___ regular food;   ___ liquid diet for 24 hours;   ___ light diet as instructed;
___ other: _____; Special Instructions: _____

WOUND CARE: ___ Keep incision clean & dry;   ___ Remove dressing at: _____ on (date) _____
___ Shower after: _____, or ___ bathe after: _____;
Other: _____
_____

CALL YOUR HEALTH CARE PROVIDER IF YOU NOTICE THE FOLLOWING SIGNS OF ILLNESS:

___ Temperature over _____ degrees F. by _____ (method);   ___ drainage from the wound;
___ Redness or swelling around the wound;   ___ opening of the incision;   ___ increasing pain;
other: _____

FOLLOW-UP CARE INSTRUCTIONS:

___ **Return to the health care provider on** _____ **at** _____
Provider phone number: _____;   ___ copy of preprinted instructions, from provider, given to patient.
___ NO APPOINTMENT, RETURN ONLY IF PROBLEMS DEVELOP.

FOR EMERGENCY PROBLEMS - CALL: _____

These discharge instructions have been explained and questions have been answered. A copy has been given to me.

Patient/Significant Other: _____ Relationship: _____
                              Signature

Nurse's signature: _____ Date: _____ ; Time: _____

---

the count basin. The nurse agreed, and the surgery was completed with the count unresolved and no further action taken.

Mr. N complained of severe abdominal pain over the next 2 days. When the pain increased instead of decreasing following surgery, the nurse caring for Mr. N contacted the surgeon. An X-ray revealed the presence of an 18-inch by 6-inch absorbent sponge in the abdominal cavity.

Another surgery was performed to remove the sponge. Mr. N suffered a pulmonary embolism during the second surgery and did not recover from the postanesthesia period.

Failure to properly follow up on an unresolved count during the initial surgery led to the need for further surgery and was found to be the indirect cause of the patient's death. Litigation pursued, and an award of $500,000 went to Mr. N's mother for wrongful death from medical and nursing malpractice.

The failure to stop a procedure when the sponge, sharp, or instrument count was unresolved was blamed on the circulating and scrub nurses. The surgeon failed to recognize the responsibility of the surgical team and the safety of the patient in discounting the nurse's report of an unresolved sponge count.

Although this is a shortened version of a case, the facts can lend themselves to an in-depth discussion of the need to follow established OR policies and protocols for the safe execution of all surgical procedures.

RECORDING PATIENT CARE IN PSYCHIATRIC/ MENTAL HEALTH NURSING

15

Sue E. Meiner

Chapter Outline

The therapeutic relationship is central to psychiatric/mental health (P/MH) nursing. This chapter presents areas of potential liability that can occur as a result of the therapeutic relationship between the nurse and the patient. It focuses on areas of recording and reporting specific interactions or interventions. The P/MH nurse's competence in determining how nursing interventions will be structured and implemented is important.

The patient's medical record must contain sufficient information to provide written communication for other members of the psychiatric team. Other reasons include confirming to insurance companies that appropriate services were provided and providing a defense for claims of nursing negligence. Avoiding ethical and legal misfeasance always must be a consideration of care in the performance of the P/MH nurse's therapeutic interactions (Woody, 1997). Table 15.1 lists the 10 most common liability issues in P/MH nursing.

LEVELS OF PSYCHIATRIC/MENTAL HEALTH NURSING PRACTICE

Liability for clinical assessment and decision making in P/MH nursing can be different for nurses with advanced education and experience in this field of practice. The following information explains the differences among nurses from various skill levels.

TABLE 15.1   10 Common Liabilities in Psychiatric/Mental Health Nursing

1. Suicide
2. Restraint injuries
3. Electroconvulsive therapy injuries
4. Breach of confidentiality
5. Failure to properly assess risk for self-injury
6. Failure to obtain informed consent
7. Failure to report patient abuse
8. Failure to refer a patient to a higher level of health care provider
9. Inadequate supervision of ancillary health care workers
10. Sexual contact with a patient

SOURCE: Adapted from Stuart and Laraia (1997, p. 172).

The specialty of P/MH nursing can be practiced by nursing professionals within a wide variation of levels of care. The American Nurses Association (ANA, 1994) defined two levels of P/MH nursing as follows:

1. The licensed registered nurse (RN) with a baccalaureate degree in nursing and demonstrated clinical skills beyond those of a new practitioner
2. The advanced practice RN with the minimum of a master's degree in nursing, knowledge in nursing theory, and clinical practice at an advanced skill level (the master's-prepared nurse with a doctoral degree in nursing or a related field practices at an advanced level as a certified specialist)

The work experience of the P/MH nurse is highly regarded in establishing a level of competence. The combination of education and experience is significant in the level of therapeutic nursing care delivered. Accountability and liability increase with each level as the P/MH nurse moves toward autonomy of practice including staff privileges with mental health care institutions or agencies.

The interplay of the P/MH nurse's practice and the patient's rights in the psychiatric setting is held to the same professional standards of care as in other nursing practice settings. Litigation is less common in this specialty but often is identified with the death of a patient by suicide. According to Beckmann's (1996) study, inadequate psychiatric nursing assessment was the most common breach of nursing standards of care, whereas injuries were heavily associated with the improper use of restraint devices.

RESTRAINT USE IN THE PSYCHIATRIC SETTING

Usually, the P/MH patient is competent to make medical decisions. At other times, the patient does not appreciate the potential for harm that could occur

TABLE 15.2 List of Observations and Recording of Physical Restraint Use

Monitor and record the following:

1. Skin condition at restraint sites
2. Color, temperature, and sensation in restrained extremities
3. Type of movement allowed as behavior permits
4. Position changes to prevent pressure ulcers or aspiration
5. Continued needs being met (hydration, nutrition, elimination, and hygiene)
6. If more than one site was restrained, the rotating release and reapplication pattern and patient response
7. Rationale and results from removal of the restraints

during some behaviors. This safeguarding of the well-being of the patient with mental illness requires an ongoing psychiatric evaluation with a regular physical assessment. At times, the P/MH nurse will need to omit medication or immediately administer a sedating medication. The act of restraining a patient to prevent harm to self or others is an area that requires a rapid and appropriate response.

A restraint is any device that limits a person's movement. Restraints can be mechanical, manual, or chemical. Mechanical restraints usually are padded leather or cloth strapping that is placed around one or more extremities and/or the trunk of the person. Manual restraint is the holding of a person by other persons to limit mobility. Chemical restraints usually are considered to be sedating medications.

As an intervention to patient behavior, restraints are used to protect the patient from self-inflicted harm or to prevent harm to others. It is not considered a first-line course of action in patient management. Less restrictive interventions are preferred and usually attempted before using restraints. An exception is when the imminent harm to self or others is too significant to lose time in exploring other avenues of behavior modification. Charting the use of physical restraints is essential. Recorded information concerning the events that preceded the need for restraints and the care taken to ensure a safe experience for the patient must be documented. Table 15.2 lists observations and recording of physical restraint use.

The American Psychiatric Association (APA; 1985) has supported several specific criteria for seclusion or restraints in psychiatric settings. Beyond previously stated reasons for using restraints, the APA recommends restraint use to prevent a serious disruption of treatment or environmental damage to the patient's physical area. When a reduction in environmental stimulation is necessary and medications are too dangerous to use as sedation, restraint might be the best action.

A patient with a known history of being combative requires a heightened alertness by the nursing staff. If a self-inflicted injury occurs or if another patient is injured due to the lack of observation by the nursing staff, then an issue of

TABLE 15.3 Charting Guidelines for Suicide Potential

---

1. Record the type of close supervision provided to the suicidal patient
    A. Record one-on-one care
    B. Record the assessment that determines when the threat of harm has passed
    C. Record the time and frequency of observations if one-on-one care is not provided
2. Record the assessment of the physical environment
    A. Record the removal of all potentially dangerous objects from the patient's room
    B. Record the careful administration of all medications to ensure that hoarding of potentially lethal drugs is not being done
    C. Record the inspection of the patient's room for stored medications
    D. Record that all exits (including windows) from the area are secured to prevent elopement or suicide from jumping out of a window or balcony

---

liability could result. Likewise, the patient lacking any historical or present indication of potential suicide or dangerous acts to self or others does not require a greater amount of observation than usually is practiced (Bernzweig, 1996).

The individual with mental illness who threatens suicide must be placed in a suicide alert mode, with recordings made of these observations. Table 15.3 provides guidelines for recording observations during a suicide potential.

CHARTING THE NURSING ASSESSMENT

The benefits of a structured documentation system provide the patient and the payer system with records that reflect accountability. Wiger (1997) described components of maintaining patient care accountability in documentation as "accurate diagnosis, concise treatment planning, case notes that follow the treatment plan, treatment reflecting the diagnosis, and documentation of the course of therapy" (p. x).

Nurses working with psychiatric patients must realize that this special needs population can present vastly different issues related to safety, environmental hazards, and constitutional rights. The ANA standards of care for P/MH nursing practice emphasize specific components of the interview. The assessment interview should be systematic, comprehensive, and continuous throughout each visit or treatment period.

The medical record must have information related to patient and family education presented by the P/MH nurse. Accurate recording of information given to the patient or the patient's family should be done as soon after the teaching session as possible. A thorough recording of the teaching session should include the patient's response to the new information presented. When the family is the focus of the teaching session, responses might need to be quoted in the medical record.

REPORTING PERTINENT
INFORMATION TO COWORKERS

In the practice of P/MH nursing, the patient's condition can change from hour to hour or from day to day during acute phases of illness. The recording of these changes is essential to complete, relevant, objective, and timely documentation. However, the reporting of abnormal responses or changes in behavior must be passed along to coworkers that might have contact with the patient. The incidence of suicide or self-injury must be discussed with staff members caring for the patient.

PROFESSIONAL ETHICS AND THE LAW

During a therapeutic interaction, a patient discusses an immediate past episode of abuse toward a child, a spouse, or an elder. Ethically, the P/MH nurse holds this communication as confidential. However, the law mandates that acts of abuse be reported to appropriate authorities. The dilemma regarding breaking the confidence of the therapeutic relationship must be tempered by the ethical standards that hold the law as supreme over ethics. If this situation is related to distant past abuse, then the gray area of reporting comes into play. The most appropriate course of action is to refer this to the supervising psychiatrist or, in the case of an advanced practice P/MH nurse, to legal counsel for clarification of the law in that jurisdiction. Any decision in this regard must be legally determined and the therapeutic preference of the practitioner (Woody, 1997).

COMMON-LAW DUTY TO WARN

In the P/MH nursing setting, there can be no assurance that the practitioner's education or experience can predict dangerous or violent behavior in an unstable patient. In this case, public policy drives the decision-making efforts. Statutes and common law rulings dictate that the practitioner errs on the cautious side instead of giving the patient the benefit of the doubt. These policies are directed at protection of the public at the expense of the rights of the patient.

Individual liability for breach of confidentiality of a therapeutic relationship is less binding than the liability caused by harm to another person or persons. In fact, case law shows that the P/MH nurse therapist is more likely to fall under liability for not communicating a timely warning.

According to Soreff and McDuffee (1993), the admission assessment helps the initiation of a therapeutic relationship between the nurse and patient and builds a firm ground for communication. The supportive relationship of the nurse toward achieving an optimal level of functioning depends greatly on information obtained during the admission assessment. JCAHO (1995) listed standards for patient care that require every patient to receive nursing care based on a documented assessment of his or her needs. In addition, the Health Care Financing Administration requires that the hospital ensure that the nursing staff develop and maintain a current nursing care plan for each patient.

The importance of documenting the behavior of a psychiatric patient is essential for informing other nurses of care given and for giving physicians an accurate 24-hour observation of the symptoms and condition of the psychiatric patient.

The problem list in the initial plan of care will need to have frequent recording of progress toward resolution. When that problem is resolved, appropriate recording of that fact must be made to end the responsibility of continuing assessment for that problem. However, if new assessment findings cause a need to reinstate a problem to the list that had been resolved previously, then the new problem will need a new problem number. All future charting on that problem will need to use the newest number. In this manner, a chronological record can be maintained on the changes to the patient's condition.

Many types of legal situations can develop in psychiatric hospitals. Following discharge, a patient might sue the physician, the nurse, or the institution for alleged mistreatment. The patient's will might be contested because of his or her mental illness. Compensation or insurance cases might arise in which all recorded materials could be very important. The P/MH nursing records often are the most valuable source of reference for verifying or disproving legal accusations. The P/MH nurse should be familiar with this aspect of patient care when engaging in documentation in the psychiatric setting.

PSYCHIATRIC HOME HEALTH CARE

The National Association for Home Care (1996) related information on the percentage of home care provided to persons with a primary psychiatric diagnosis. Their percentage was a mere 3.4%. However, the actual number can be identified only when secondary diagnosis of mental disorders is analyzed.

The transitions from institutionalization to community mental health programs have continued to increase throughout the United States. With the addition of Medicare reimbursement for psychiatric home care and a trend toward less restrictive treatment of mental disorders, the outlook for psychiatric home care is positive (Stuart and Laraia, 1997).

With the change in setting from an outpatient or professional office to the patient's home, certain conditions for therapy are modified. These issues are cultural sensitivity, flexibility of interaction boundaries, trust, and safety concerns for the psychiatric home health nurse (Stuart and Laraia, 1997).

The cultural sensitivity issues that may face the P/MH nurse in the home setting include the family hierarchy and family members' reaction to mental illness. It may be affected by prejudices related to health care and alternative therapy involvement by the patient or family members.

Boundary issues may involve the sharing of home rituals to build a therapeutic relationship. An example might be sharing in a family celebration by eating a piece of cake and having a cup of coffee or tea. This is not considered improper nurse-patient behavior.

The trust factor is central to the success of home care. The nurse trusts the patient to continue the plan of care between visits, whereas the patient trusts that the nurse will be clinically sound and reliable. The safety concern arises when a possibility for aggressive behavior or the potential for suicide exists. The nursing care plan needs to have an acceptable plan for emergent problems (Stuart and Laraia, 1997).

Often, the P/MH home care nurse works as a member of the home health care team. The clear and understandable recording of mental health care goals is essential for ongoing psychiatric home care. Accountability for continued assessment emphasizing outcome-oriented care should be the goal of the nurse practicing in this special area of P/MH nursing. Maintaining an open communication with the primary care physician or psychiatrist is vitally important to support the home care maintenance of the patient (Daudell-Strejc and Murphy, 1995).

CONCLUSION

Restraint issues are quite commonplace in the psychiatric setting. Their use, and the documentation associated with their use, is essential to avoid injury to the patient. The recording of the monitoring and ongoing assessment can prevent claims of false imprisonment or injury from the use of restraints after a P/MH patient is discharged from the facility.

Records that note specific suicidal precautions must clarify the nurse's actions. If the nurse fails to detain or restrain a patient or omits medication that would have prevented a patient from harming himself or herself or others, then liability for malpractice could result if the outcome of the omission is injuries or even suicide.

Patient and family education must be recorded in the medical record. Accurate reporting is an element of nursing care that should be done when time allows, following a patient event. Prompt and thorough recording of the event and the outcome is essential in P/MH nursing.

The specialty of P/MH nursing is guided by the Standards of Psychiatric/Mental Health Clinical Nursing Practice, as set by the ANA (1994). Nurses preparing to work in this area or nurses with P/MH experience need to review these standards regularly to ensure that the care rendered to patients in their care meets the standards of practice.

CASE STUDY

Mrs. K, a 42-year-old woman, was admitted to the closed psychiatric unit with suicidal precautions. Her depression had continued to increase over the past 3 months in spite of medication and psychotherapy. After 5 days, she seemed less depressed and was moved to another closed unit with fewer restrictions related to movement throughout the unit.

A day room, activities room, dining room, nursing station, and semiprivate sleeping room were available for each patient to visit at will during specific hours. A multistall bathroom was located off the activities room. The bathroom was locked unless a psychiatric aide was present to accompany a patient.

The P/MH nurse completed an assessment of Mrs. K. The findings included concern that she was feeling well enough to act on her suicidal thoughts. The nurse recommended that she be returned to a more restrictive environment until less danger of suicide was evident.

The psychologist visited the patient shortly after the nurse's assessment. When the nurse discussed her findings with the psychologist, she was told that the improvement in Mrs. K's mood was genuine and that she was getting better and needed fewer restrictions instead of more observation.

The nurse charted her assessment but failed to record the difference in opinion that had occurred between the two professionals. The psychologist was interrupted in the visit to the unit and had to leave before dictating her visit and findings.

At bed check, Mrs. K could not be found, and she had not been seen for more than 2 hours. The bathroom attached to the activities room was found unlocked, and Mrs. K was found hanging from the curtain rod by a bed sheet taken from her bed. She was pronounced dead at the scene with an estimated time of death of approximately 60 to 90 minutes before the discovery of her body.

The responsibility of patient care, as determined by a P/MH nurse following an assessment, requires that appropriate nursing judgments be made and appropriate interventions implemented. When changes in a patient's physical or mental condition are assessed, a nursing action must follow. If the decision is not to act but rather to observe further, then that is an action. That decision must be shown in the patient's record.

The outcome of this case involved a dispute regarding the verbal communication between the nurse and the psychologist. The case was settled out of court, with an undisclosed amount of compensation going to Mrs. K's family.

COMMUNICATIONS IN COMMUNITY AND HOME HEALTH CARE NURSING

16

Sue E. Meiner
With Nancy Kuhrik
and Marilee Kuhrik

Chapter Outline

This chapter presents information related to the variety of health care settings in which licensed nurses practice within the urban or rural community. The roles are as varied as the titles. Each role has special needs and/or a special policy for recording information about the patients who receive the services. The term *distributive nursing* often is used to refer to those areas of nursing that relate to services rendered to individuals with or without the component of illness. Broad titles included within this context are the public health nurse, the community health nurse, the school nurse, the occupational health nurse (OHN), the home health nurse, and the parish nurse. The settings are described under the heading for each specialty, and a section on the health fair is included at the end of the chapter.

FEDERAL LAWS, STATUTES, AND COMMUNITY-BASED NURSING

Public health nursing has been around since the early 1900s in New York City, where the visiting nurse provided the main health care for indigent immigrant families in slum dwellings (Kalisch and Kalisch, 1984). From this beginning in America, public health nursing and community nursing have provided a safety net for those persons and families unable to care for or understand their health needs. The Social Security Act of 1935 provided for the general welfare of the elderly, many classifications of disabled persons, maternal and child health, and public health (Guido, 1997).

In 1944, the Public Health Service Act brought together all the existing public health programs under one law. The meaning of the term *public health* changed from health care delivered to the public at large to an identified group of services that would be available to everyone. The funding would combine federal and state sources. The administration of these services would be at the federal and state agency levels.

Services have expanded and now include family planning services; migrant workers' health services; prevention and control of heart disease and stroke; programs specific to cancer, kidney disease, sickle cell anemia, diabetes, and sudden infant death syndrome; and funding of a variety of research and educational programs. The National Institutes of Health were established through this consolidation.

In 1965, Medicare and Medicaid were added to the federally funded programs for the health and welfare of citizens of the United States. Several additions to each of these programs have occurred over the past decades. Programs for alcohol detoxification, hospice care, and medical reimbursement through Medicare Part B have evolved (Guido, 1997).

COMMUNITY NURSING

Community nursing encompasses far more than overseeing community health care. This specialty consists of public health nursing, community health nursing, school nursing, occupational nursing, and parish nursing. The term used by Miller (1990) described the major purpose of public and community health nursing as health care pertaining to aggregates. This larger number of patients is the main difference between the community nurse and the home care nurse.

The former cares for a community of persons, whereas the latter cares primarily for one patient within a family setting.

SCHOOL HEALTH NURSING

The nonmedical environment of the school health nurse requires implementing independent judgment related to student health and welfare issues. Emergency care and treatment skills were essential requirements for school nurses prior to the emergency response services of paramedics in the 1970s. Many of these skills still are needed in rapid assessment of children with traumatic injuries or when an illness occurs that necessitates immediate medical attention. Regardless of the paramedic services available to the school district, the school nurse must be competent to provide a standard of care that a reasonably prudent nurse working in an emergency setting would provide. This standard was upheld in Minnesota case law when the court ruled that school nurses have a higher duty of care than hospital nurses to make an assessment for emergency medical care (*Schlussler v. Independent School District No. 200 et al.*, 1989).

OCCUPATIONAL HEALTH NURSING

As nurses have entered industry as employee health advocates, the liability issues have increased as well. Much of the increase in the quantity and complexity of occupational health nurses' (OHN) work has resulted from Occupational Safety and Health Administration (OSHA) laws, mandatory reporting laws, and workers' compensation laws. OSHA has the duty to protect American workers from hazards recognized in specific industries. It is the enforcing agency for the Centers for Disease Control's guidelines for tuberculosis prevention and blood-borne pathogen exposure in work sites. The OHN, under most situations of industry, is given the responsibility for overseeing these programs.

The role of the OHN is varied, depending on the industry or work setting. However, documentation must include areas that are required by law and by health needs. Developing and implementing safety programs within the work setting is one mandatory area of performance. The programs must follow requirements set by local, state, and/or federal guidelines. OSHA standards are rigidly enforced. Documentation of safety and health promotion efforts need to be in writing and placed in a designated area for review by inspection teams from these overseeing agencies (OSHA, 1970).

Ongoing safety programs and drills with community fire and rescue departments are other areas of accountability in most industrial settings. A protocol for rapid assessment and appropriate (type of rescue vehicle, timeliness, and backup medical support) transport of injured workers must be provided in writing and available to all occupational nurses at each site. Other responsibilities exist for supervising first aid responders and for equipment. In many work settings, the OHN carries the responsibility of teaching first aid to nonmedical personnel. Duties include ensuring availability of equipment that might be needed in the event of an emergency situation. Potential liability could exist if inadequate, outdated, and/or ineffective first aid equipment is present when an accident occurs.

Written Protocols for Urgent Care Versus Emergency Care

Specific guidelines and protocols for urgent care versus emergency care are needed in written format and must be available for inspection by licensing agencies and for in-service education. The written protocols are for the delivery of nursing interventions following nursing assessments that fall under each state's Nurse Practice Act. Open or loose guidelines can result in the charge of practicing medicine without a license. This places the liability of malpractice on the OHN's shoulders.

Occupational Health Nursing Reports

Workers' compensation claims frequently are followed by the OHN. The initial file must have documentation related to the job-related injury including emergency actions taken by the employee and the OHN. The written report will become the first in a long chain of paper trails if any of the parties do not agree with the circumstances of the accident or the immediate follow-up actions.

Documentation coordination for all health care disciplines may become the exclusive role of the OHN. Accurate records are needed that state the date, time, discipline involved, and employee response. Periodic reports must be submitted to the insurance carrier for reimbursement and to continue the employee's workers' compensation claim. Documentation should include information that substantiates that the services were reasonable and necessary to the recovery of the employee.

HOME HEALTH CARE

Discharge of the patient very soon after a major health deviation, major surgery, treatment for trauma, or regulation of lifesaving pharmacotherapeutics is the standard in the late 1990s. Sending the patient home for continued follow-up care releases the patient from the facility much earlier than in previous decades. This decrease in the length of acute care time is evolving into a higher acuity rate for home care patients.

The factors that affect the licensed nurse's role in documentation of home care have increased steadily as controls by regulatory agencies have escalated. The overseeing state agencies have set standards for maintaining the clinical record of home care patients. Medicare and Medicaid have added requirements of verification of skilled services done by licensed nursing personnel prior to reimbursement. JCAHO (1993) has set standards for voluntary accreditation of agencies that deliver health care services at home. Documentation review is a key matter in certification of home health care (HHC) agencies (Marrelli, 1994).

ADEQUATE AND ACCURATE
DOCUMENTATION OF RECORDS

Documentation is a time-consuming but necessary part of the community and home care nurse's obligation. This obligation is professional, legal, and financial. The home care record must reflect all of the care, teaching, and other interactions that take place during a visit. This includes information to and from patients, family members, significant others, physicians, medical supply services, pharmacy, and all other health-related support services that come into the home setting. The accuracy of the actual content of the home care record should be objective rather than subjective, and terms used need to be measurable rather than approximate (Marrelli, 1994).

Proper monitoring instructions in documentation are vital. The legal implications can become quite significant if safety instructions are not recorded and an accident occurs in the home while using equipment that was obtained by, and initial instructions were given by, the home care nurse.

Telephone Orders

Physician contact often is made by telephone and/or mail. The physician must certify that a plan of care is appropriate for each patient to obtain reimbursement from insurance companies, independent health care plans, and government programs such as Medicare. The plan of care usually is done at the time of discharge from an acute care or extended care facility. The home care agency receives the referral with basic information related to the patient's diagnosis, an established plan of care, medications, follow-up visits to the physician, and any special needs or considerations specific to that patient.

The home care nurse often arrives at the patient's home and immediately identifies needs that had not been anticipated at discharge. Although the patient must be under the care of a physician, the home care nurse works very independently of direct medical supervision. Immediate interventions are needed when discharge planning has failed to include essential elements of home care needs. The most frequent action taken by a home care nurse in this situation is to make a telephone call to the physician for additional orders. Obtaining telephone orders always is risky in that communication might be brief, incomplete, or confusing. Special attention must be focused on telephone orders. First, the nurse needs to ensure that both parties on the telephone are discussing the same patient. Repetition and clarification are necessary if the nurse is unclear as to what the physician has ordered. If the order does not provide an intervention that seems appropriate for the patient's needs or problem, then it should be questioned, with the specific needs being reiterated (Lovejoy, 1997; Marrelli, 1994).

When telephone orders are taken by the home care nurse, the most prudent routine is to repeat the orders in their entirety to ensure total accuracy, beginning with the patient's name, date, and time, the orders received, and the physician's name. Spelling medication names and medical equipment names is strongly recommended given that many words sound alike. Some equipment orders, including those for oxygen supplies and the amount to be delivered per mask or cannula, need repeating for clarification. Oxygen should be considered as a medication with the same strict adherence to the manner in which any medication is administered.

The order sheet must have the physician's signature within a specified time interval set according to the home care agency's policy for verbal orders. Remember that all telephone orders must be countersigned by the ordering physician. Without this signature, the home care nurse could be held liable for injury to the patient or, in some states, for practicing beyond a nursing license and scope of practice (Humphrey and Milone-Nuzzo, 1996).

Basic Home Care Documentation

In the home care record, pertinent information can include things such as distances in the home setting for documenting ambulation and mobility issues. Comments made by the patient and/or family members related to care issues are essential to include in the written record. The information needs to be objectively stated rather than reflective of the nurse's data interpretation. For example, it would be incorrect to document the following: "Mrs. Smith is not in a good mood. She seems upset because her family is not visiting her very often." A more correct form for reporting this objective situation would be the following: "Mrs. Smith is sitting in her living room crying. When asked by this nurse why she is upset, she stated, "My family has deserted me. They never come to see me anymore." The first charting example is presumptuous on the part of the nurse. The second example is objectively stated and identifies the patient's stated feelings (rather than the nurse's interpretation of the patient's behavior) using the patient's own words (Foreman, 1993).

Cleanliness of the home (or lack thereof), especially surrounding the patient's environment, is important to document. Universal precautions are required when body fluids pose a health hazard to others in the home environment. When oxygen is required, a backup system needs to be made available for emergency needs in the event of an untimely oxygen supply depletion.

Documenting the Plan of Care

The nurse always must check charting to make sure that it has stated relevant care determined by planned interventions. All assessments need to match the plan of care. To prevent redundant charting, the data must be clear, concise, and devoid of abbreviations that can have several meanings. The use of approved abbreviations is essential for clarity. Other components include legible writing and correct spelling and should include any specific precautions that other members of the health care team might need to know during their visits.

Whenever possible, preprinted flow sheets should be developed for routine elements of care. Diagrams for noting skin conditions, surgical wounds, pressure ulcers, and areas of pain or to document other findings that are more appropriate to diagrams should be used. The body diagram should show a front, side, and back view. This form can be used with many headings (Goldrick and Larson, 1993; Springhouse, 1997). See Chart 14.2 for an example.

Specific Health Deviations

Documenting Pain

A heading for documenting areas of pain and using numbers that correspond to a pain scale will send a very specific message to the other health care team members who visit at other times. This system can provide a rapid review of previous care that will need to be reevaluated on future visits. When the presence of pain is noted, an action statement or intervention plan is absolutely necessary. This plan or intervention must have an outcome evaluation identified. If family or home caregivers instructions are explicit, then these need to be included in the documentation on instructions or teaching.

Always include a final comment on the teaching-learning process. Check to be sure that the recipient of the information being taught did understand and/or return a demonstration to indicate that what was taught was learned. It is important to document the nature of that teaching session. Note the name of the person receiving the information and the person's relationship to the patient.

Documenting Skin Care and Wounds

The clinical home health record (CHHR) will benefit from the use of photographs (with the patient's permission) of any wounds that are being treated. The initial photograph will serve as documentation for the record and for purposes of reimbursement by most third-party payers. As the wound heals or does not heal, additional pictures will need to be added to the record, shown to the physician, and possibly sent to the reimbursement agency for continued treatment. However, the photograph cannot replace a written description of the wound, the total care given in detail, and all instructions and supplies that are in the possession of the patient or caregivers.

When training is necessary for wound care, allow time for a return demonstration prior to leaving the home. Then document the time, the potential to successfully perform the task, and quality of the return demonstration by the patient or caregiver. Written instructions are better than verbal directions for most wound care problems. In any event, charting who followed the instructions and how they were followed is important.

Other methods of documenting a pressure ulcer or wound include a sheet of paper with the front and back drawing of an outline of the human body. Mark the location of the wound on the body form. Attempt to draw the form or shape of the actual wound. Label the shape with a number and record information related to that site after that number on the page (Goldrick and Larson, 1993) (Table 16.1).

Information that is pertinent is the stage, size, drainage, and characteristics of the wound. While noting the size of the wound, include width, height, and depth. If these measurements are irregular, then note them using map coordinates of north to south and east to west. Equally important, note redness, edema, and odor. Finally, note that a drawing has been marked and is an attachment to the main body of nurses notes. Paginate and date all notes for this visit, and include the patient's name and identification number. The initials and/or name of the nurse must be clearly readable.

Recording Physician or Physician's Office Staff Contacts

Health care team members rely heavily on the CHHR for essential information related to the patient's current state of health, treatments being implemented, and other interventions. These records should contain information related to any change in the patient's condition, in medications being taken, or in any refill information that will maintain pharmacotherapeutics per the physician's orders. Documenting all contact with the physician, time, subject discussed, content of that exchange (e.g., a status report and orders received), and identification of the time for the physician's next update is essential. Specific notation of the intended contact by the physician will need to be clear. State if

TABLE 16.1 An Example of Wound Care Documentation

The following brief statements are examples of documentation that identify professional skills in wound management through home care (each statement is an independent example):

1. Systems assessment of the patient with a Stage III, 2.5 cm × 3.0 cm, 1.0 cm deep, right hip pressure ulcer
2. Skilled observation and assessment of healing process/signs of infection
3. Patient and caregiver teaching of wound irrigation and dressing technique to be done once in the late morning and once at bedtime at night, daily
4. Wound irrigated w/ hydrogen peroxide, flushed w/ sterile normal saline solution, open packages form sterile field, use sterile gloves, pack w/ sterile iodoform gauze (20 inches), use sterile Q-tips, cover with two 4×4's, and topped w/ one 6×6 ABD pad (use sterile gloves, Q-tips, and scissors)
5. Evaluate patient's response to treatments and interventions, and report untoward responses or reactions to the physician as necessary
6. Assess patient for nutrition and hydration status
7. Plan future contacts with patient and leave written plan of care for caregivers to follow that includes instructions for reporting abnormal events or any changes in the patient's health condition

and when a physician's office visit is to be scheduled. If the office staff of the physician states that a return call will be made, then note that information as well. Future contact with the physician may be by telephone, by specific instructions to be mailed to the patient, or by a personal visit to the patient's home. If this information is given to the home care nurse, then it must be recorded in a note specified as communication with the physician or doctor's office staff.

Differences Between Acute Care Records and Home Care Records

The CHHR has some differences when compared to the hospital medical record. This record is the only written source for communications among the HHC team (Eggland, 1996). The CHHR is the primary foundation for an evaluation of the care given to the patient and additional instructions for care that are given to the family. Although this source is primarily for reference to other team members, it also serves to inform and support reimbursement matters with third-party payers. Faulty documentation can lead to a denial of payment for the services provided.

Teaching and training of the patient and family or regular caregiver must be documented at the end of the visit. Any information, flyers, or notes that were left for the family to review or to use to contact a specific member of the HHC team will need to be recorded in the record. Names of persons in the home who

TABLE 16.2 Guidelines for Effective Documentation

---

1. The medical record must be readable. When handwritten records are kept, write or print neatly and legibly.
2. Use dark ink colors unless your agency has specific colors for different charting purposes.
3. Start every entry with the date and time.
4. Use only accepted abbreviations that are identified in your agency's procedures or skills manual. Do not use slang words or phrases. Remain objective and nonjudgmental in *all* charting in the medical record.
5. End every entry with your name and title or your initials with your name printed elsewhere on the same page accompanied by those same initials for identification.
6. Describe all care, teaching, or other interventions provided. Do not omit a care area because you think that it is expected or routine.
7. Describe the patient's response to the activities provided. When family members are involved, describe their responses to all activities in which they were included.
8. Maintain a consecutive and chronological order to all written notes.
9. Use patient, family, or caregiver statements whenever possible. Quotes are preferred over paraphrasing. Be accurate about the times and the services provided.
10. Do not skip any lines or leave gaps in the record. Never leave space for someone else to record notes when they are not able to write their own activities unless you state that you observed the care (name the person providing services) being given.
11. Complete notes as soon as possible after the services are provided. If the patient's home is not conducive to writing in the record, then stop as soon as possible after leaving the home to complete the notes.

SOURCE: Adapted from Marrelli (1994).

are assuming responsibility for care or oversight between home care visits will need to be placed in the home care record. Table 16.2 lists guidelines for effective documentation.

Accident or Incident Reports in Home Care

When an accident occurs within the home care setting, an incident report is necessary. Remember that the person who witnessed the incident or was the first one on the scene to discover the occurrence can sign a report as firsthand information. If the nurse is not the first person on the scene, then the facts need to be written as given in quotation format with the name of the reporter clearly identified. Record the details in objective terms only and do not add assumptions to any report. If a fall is witnessed, then it must be reported as it was observed. The objective form would be to report the following: "Patient found on floor beside chair." Then the report is continued with an assessment and interventions. Descriptions of the actions taken with the patient and any instructions given to the patient or caregivers need to be included. Each agency has a policy and a procedure for completing incident reports.

CONTINUOUS QUALITY
IMPROVEMENT IN HOME CARE

Quality initiatives have proliferated in all health care settings over the past decade. Continuous quality improvement has been adopted to serve as the foundation to keep pace with changes in health care delivery, personnel requirements and expectations, and supportive administration policies (Foreman, 1993).

WHEN HOME CARE PATIENTS COMPLAIN

Documentation of patient complaints must be followed with an action message based on the immediate follow-up of the concern. The problem should be reported to the supervisor or manager as soon as possible. Recording conversations between the home care nurse and the supervisor should be a part of the record. Use professional judgment regarding all written or verbal communication with patients, their families, and involved coworkers.

PARISH NURSING AND THE NEED
FOR RECORD KEEPING

Parish nurses are either volunteers or employees of a church ministry. In some cases, a parish nurse (PN) has a joint appointment between a local medical center and the religious congregation. Dunkel (1996) defined the PN as a registered professional nurse who provides holistic nursing services to members of a congregation while working with community health providers.

The PN assumes many roles including those of educator, volunteer coordinator, referral agent, and (at times) family advocate for special needs. Regardless of the role being performed, and despite the fact that the PN does not normally perform hands-on nursing care, careful documentation needs to be made. A major issue for the PN is the maintenance of confidentiality of services rendered and the documentation of care. A secured, locked file drawer should be available to the PN for keeping parishioner records of counseling, health care referrals, and personal information that must be included in parish medical records. Breach of confidentiality can place the PN in a position of liability. The type of records that need to be kept for future reference and for the protection of the PN from potential litigation is illustrated in the following example.

The PN counsels a parishioner to go to an emergency room or to call a primary care provider regarding a significantly elevated blood pressure taken during a home visit. The parishioner promises the PN that she will follow up on the PN's advice by calling her son and daughter to take her to the hospital. She wants to do it privately so that she can say personal things to her children. She assures the PN that this will be done as soon as their visit is over. The parishioner does not comply with her promise to follow up on the elevated blood pressure. That night, she suffers a severe stroke.

The parishioner's family members are angry that the PN did not call an ambulance, call a relative, or stay with the parishioner until the PN was sure that her advice had been heeded. No record was made on the advice or reaction/response of the parishioner. The only record was a blood pressure card recording the severely elevated blood pressure and signed by the PN. The liability issue here depends on many factors. However, the need for documenting on permanently retained records could have provided information that might have explained the PN's actions more fully.

HEALTH FAIRS AND NURSING DOCUMENTATION

Licensed nurses are asked to respond annually to appeals for volunteers at local health fairs throughout the United States. These events usually provide basic health screening for individuals who do not see primary care providers on a regular basis. This might be due to a lack of health care insurance or a lack of convenience. No matter the reason, most tests done during a health fair are free.

In preparation for the health fair, the nurse determines whether a fire and safety plan is in place where the fair will be held. If so, then this plan should be reviewed by the nurse and all providers in the fair. If no plan is in place, then the nurse should locate the emergency exits, telephones, fire extinguishers, and other emergency equipment. All doors, phones, and equipment will need to be clearly identified by signage and instruction sheets for all providers. Biohazard materials (sharps) boxes need to be distributed and their locations marked on the fair map.

The screenings done usually consist of height; weight; vital signs (blood pressure, pulse, respiratory rate, and sometimes temperature); some basic and noninvasive cancer screening and information; nutrition and special diet information; cholesterol and blood glucose checks; oral and dental screening; basic respiratory function tests; screening of the feet for fungus, deformities, and proper shoe fitting; and other screening tests.

The nurse records the results of specific tests such as routine information on vital signs, rapid blood test readings, respiratory and nutritional findings, and other information specific to the variety of testing being done at that health fair. Depending on the policy of the agency sponsoring the health fair to the public, written instructions might be provided for follow-up by the participant. A copy of these instructions can be maintained for a 30-month period by the sponsoring agency. In the event of an unexpected contact by a lawyer, the copy might prove valuable in determining the final instructions given to the health fair participant.

CONCLUSION

The unique setting of community, distributive, or home care nursing frequently places the licensed nurse in a position of autonomy in decision making. The nurse assumes the responsibility for coordination of a wide variety of services to patients who might not be seen by a physician for extended periods of time. Decisions regarding treatment applications, health promotion, illness management, and cost containment are intertwined throughout the professional services that are rendered. Priorities of care and documentation are essential for continuity of services from other coordinated health care disciplines. Patient and family education is a fundamental component of community and home care when an expectation of family involvement is present.

The very nature of community, distributive, and home care nursing is in a dynamic evolution. Changes in rules, regulations, government programs, third-party payer concerns, and liability issues are a constant reality. The role of documentation in these practice settings is the only source of communication that is available to other members of the health care team. Therefore, the care plan usually is based on the documentation of each member of the team, with the community/home care nurse providing the cornerstone of communication.

CASE STUDY

At 84 years of age, Mr. K was a home care patient living with his widowed daughter-in-law in her home. The daughter-in-law's employment necessitated her leaving the home at 9:30 p.m. and returning home by 8:30 a.m. During this time, Mr. K was alone in the home.

After a physician's office visit, an HHC nurse was ordered to begin home visits three times a week due to several small Stage II pressure ulcers on Mr. K's coccyx and right ischial spine. He had lost 15 pounds since the previous visit (6 months earlier). The home care was to include teaching Mrs. K (the daughter-in-law) about skin care, positioning, mobility, and nutritional needs.

After several visits, the HHC nurse recorded that a plan of teaching had been implemented and that the Stage II pressure ulcers were nearly healed. A note was sent to the physician to report the closing of the case. When the physician received the note, another call was made for a weekly assessment for skin and nutritional condition for 1 month.

The HHC nurse assigned to the area in which Mr. K lived had a full home care assignment and accepted Mr. K's case because it required very little time. The next two weekly visits were recorded as the pressure areas returning as Stage I and then Stage II. On the third weekly visit, two Stage III and four Stage II pressure ulcers were assessed. Mr. K appeared to be dehydrated and was unclean and unshaven. On the fourth weekly visit (at 30 days), the nurse found Mr. K to be lying in urine, wearing the same pajamas from the week before (identified by a food stain on the front of the pajama top), and looking very pale and thin. No weight was obtained because he was too weak to stand on the bathroom scale.

The nurse instructed Mrs. K to call the physician and request a home health aid to help with Mr. K's physical and nutritional care. A note was made in the home care records related to these instructions. The nurse assisted Mrs. K with Mr. K's personal care and linen changing and then left the home. A discharge note was sent to the physician related to the teaching on the last visit, with the statement that the skin care was to be continued by the daughter-in-law. Although the assessments were clearly recorded in the record, the note to the physician did not discuss the increase in number and size of the pressure ulcers. The unclean condition of Mr. K and the apparent weight loss found on the last visit also were omitted.

Two weeks later, the police notified the physician about Mr. K's death and the poor condition of his body. Paramedics had arrived at the home after Mrs. K called "911" to report that Mr. K would not wake up. He had large open pressure ulcers over both hips and most boney prominences of the spine. He appeared too thin for his height and was lying in filth.

The state charged Mrs. K with neglect and elder abuse. A daughter of Mr. K's who was living in another state filed charges against the physician and home care agency, accusing the HHC nurse of nursing negligence.

The physician eventually was dismissed from the suit, but the nurse was charged with several counts of breach of standards of care. The nurse carried private malpractice insurance. Her insurance company settled the case for an unknown sum.

Failure to inform the physician of the decline in the patient's physical condition was significant in this case. Failure to assess a potential for abuse by neglect provided the plaintiff's attorney with damaging information. The home care agency had social services that were not contacted by the nurse. No follow-up was made to determine whether additional services were involved in home care.

DOCUMENTATION IN EXTENDED AND LONG-TERM CARE NURSING

17

Sue E. Meiner

Chapter Outline

Most residents in extended and long-term care (E/LTC) facilities need general supervision for health maintenance or rehabilitation. Some have very limited remaining life spans due to disease or longevity. Safeguarding daily care and activities, and promoting the best quality of life for the residents' remaining life spans, is a major goal. To attain this goal, personal assistance or reminders to perform activities of daily living become a paramount need.

Some elderly residents are cognitively impaired and are unable to do tasks of daily living without total assistance. These residents cannot understand or protect themselves from substandard or inadequate care. Family members or friends can call "hotlines" that protect confined elderly residents from E/LTC abuses or neglect. The hotline calls are acted on by inspectors from state agencies supervised by the state's Division of Aging.

Recording nursing care in E/LTC facilities requires completion of multiple complex forms that must be completed within specific time frames. With Medicare providing most of the reimbursement to these facilities, charting must follow the systems that have been established specifically for the nursing home industry. These mandatory forms are quite complex and lengthy, resulting in a time-consuming effort beginning when the resident enters the E/LTC facility.

This detailed and complex charting system provides immediate information pertaining to a resident's plan of care and the manner in which it will be, or is being, implemented. In addition, the changes in the charting systems were made in response to issues of quality of care. These changes were needed to regulate an industry identified with human rights abuse and reimbursement dilemmas.

OVERSIGHT OF LONG-TERM CARE FACILITIES

Most of the funding for long-term care (LTC) comes from the federal government. The funding is mainly through reimbursement of cost of services from Medicare and/or Medicaid.

Nursing home standards were enacted after Medicare and Medicaid came into existence. The U.S. Department of Health, Education, and Welfare headed the authority for regulation. The name was changed to the U.S. Department of Health and Human Services (DHHS), but the responsibility for nursing home regulation remains. The strict regulatory control imposed by the federal government continues to evolve and effect the quality of services and the reimbursement for nursing home services.

Health Care Financing Administration

A branch of DHHS charged with overseeing the operations of Medicare- and Medicaid-funded institutions is the Health Care Financing Administration (HCFA). In order to comply with HCFA regulations, every facility is required to complete specific documentation forms on each newly admitted resident. The Minimum Data Set for Resident Assessment and Care Screening (MDS, Version 2.0) is a set of forms. As a result of this set of forms, additional forms may be automatically triggered by a scoring system on the MDS (HCFA, 1995).

The MDS 2.0 must be completed within 14 days of the resident's admission to the facility, reviewed every 3 months, and redone if there is any significant change in the resident's condition. These forms also must be redone if the resident is transferred to an acute care setting and, on return, has a significant change. In addition to the MDS, an annual comprehensive assessment of the resident must be completed (HCFA, 1995).

TABLE 17.1 Major Regulatory Areas of the Omnibus Budget Reconciliation Act of 1987

1. Resident rights
2. Admission, transfer, and discharge rights
3. Resident behavior and facility practices
4. Quality of life
5. Resident assessment
6. Nursing services
7. Dietary services
8. Physician services
9. Specialized rehabilitative services
10. Central services
11. Pharmacy services
12. Infection control
13. Physical environment
14. Administration

Omnibus Budget Reconciliation Act

In 1987, Congress imposed dozens of new requirements on E/LTC facilities through the Omnibus Budget Reconciliation Act (OBRA). Under the three provisions of the OBRA, the provision of service requirement included quality of care for nursing home residents. The OBRA ushered in a new phase of professional accountability for the care of older persons in nursing homes. The results of this act established the requirement of documenting a comprehensive assessment within 14 days of every resident's admission to an E/LTC facility, which in turn is charted on the MDS 2.0 forms. To complete the documentation requirements, a comprehensive plan of care, based on the nursing assessment, must be completed within 7 days of completion of the MDS assessment. However, a care plan needs to be developed to meet the immediate needs of the resident based on an initial nursing assessment. This comprehensive assessment and plan of care also must be reviewed every 3 months, repeated annually, and changed with any significant alteration in the resident's condition (HCFA, 1989). Table 17.1 lists the major regulatory elements of the OBRA.

Medicare and Medicaid

Because Medicare and Medicaid provide the majority of the funding for LTC services, they have eligibility requirements that must be followed to receive reimbursement. Medicare provides reimbursements for skilled care and has stricter documentation requirements concerning the care rendered. Medicare requires a revised care plan with a change in the resident's health status and ongoing documentation for new or continued care.

Medicaid requires documentation relating to the care being received by the resident, with a revised plan of care, and with any change in status. Both Medicare and Medicaid require monthly resident reevaluations with documentation of expected outcomes according to the plan of care.

FORMS OF DOCUMENTATION

The Minimum Data Set

The MDS 2.0 is mandated by OBRA and must be completed on every resident. Areas contained in the MDS are identified by sections with numbered subsections. This instrument is intended to be an interdisciplinary assessment tool. The social worker, dietician, and activity specialists are required to complete appropriate sections of the initial evaluation instrument. Each facility must stipulate which sections are to be completed by other members of the health care team. Due to the timeliness issues related to completing the forms, nurses can complete all sections unless facility policy dictates exceptions.

The MDS 2.0 also must be revised when there is a significant change in the resident's physical or mental condition. It must be reviewed every 3 months and repeated annually, with appropriate recording of these events. The MDS forms provide a foundation for identification of indicators and descriptors that can trigger attention concerning a specific health problem. This information, combined with the Resident Assessment Protocol (RAP), leads to an effective care plan (Foltz, 1994; HCFA, 1994, 1995).

The Resident Assessment Protocol

The RAP summary is another mandated document by federal regulation. Along with the MDS 2.0, the RAP provides clinical practice guidelines and additional insight necessary for a comprehensive assessment. The primary function of the RAP is to promote the resident's highest possible level of functioning. This form must be completed within 14 days of admission. It is an 18-item problem-oriented instrument. The RAP also must be reviewed and updated or amended through the 21st day of residency in the facility (HCFA, 1995). Table 17.2 lists the clinical areas addressed by both the MDS and the RAP.

Plan of Care Using the Minimum Data Set

An initial plan of care must be completed by the nurse on the patient's admission to an LTC facility. After completion of the MDS 2.0 and the RAP,

TABLE 17.2 Clinical Areas Addressed by the Minimum Data Set and the Resident Assessment Protocol

1. Delirium
2. Cognitive loss/dementia
3. Visual function
4. Communication
5. Activities of daily living function/rehabilitation potential
6. Urinary incontinence/indwelling catheter/bowel function
7. Psychosocial well-being
8. Mood state
9. Behavior problems
10. Activities
11. Falls
12. Dental care
13. Pressure ulcers
14. Nutritional status
15. Feeding tubes
16. Dehydration/fluid maintenance
17. Psychotropic drug use
18. Physical restraint

changes to the plan of care might need to be made to provide for any areas that were triggered during the MDS and RAP assessment phases. The plan of care also should be reviewed at least every 3 months or when there is any significant change with the resident (HCFA, 1995).

The care planning process should include any family members who desire to participate in the ongoing care of the resident. Certified nursing assistants (CNAs) provide most of the care in LTC facilities. Therefore, they are an integral part of the planning process and, as such, should be included in each care planning session.

COMMON DOCUMENTATION PROBLEMS

Common Problems With Individualized Care Plans

The MDS 2.0 and the RAP have a 14-day completion date. It is imperative that any care plan that is done be reassessed after the completion of the MDS and the RAP. Additional care areas often are identified that require changing or modifying the original plan of care.

During the survey process or during litigation, the care plan is scrutinized for completeness and timing. The care plan must reflect changes in the patient's condition and treatment goals. An important concept to remember in evaluating a care plan is that the set goals must be attainable and unique to the individual resident's needs (HCFA, 1995).

Supervision of Certified Nursing Assistant Charting Activities

CNAs are responsible for most of the basic nursing care, or assisted care, given to residents. The licensed nurse is responsible for supervising CNAs. Supervision includes observing to determine whether assignments are completed and correctly recorded. When flow sheets are incomplete, doubt exists as to completion of any missing items of care. The licensed nurse has the responsibility of making sure that residents receive the care that is written on their care plans.

Incomplete flow sheets, or those completed in areas of care that could not possibly have been done, provide a target for speculation in the event of a negligence claim. When records indicate that care was given at a time when the patient was out of the facility, an immediate investigation related to this deficiency is mandated by the chief nurse of the facility. An example of this scenario can be the charting of eating a meal by percentage of food taken while the resident was miles away in an outpatient office having a diagnostic test.

Charting errors can occur when nursing care is recorded at the end of the tour of duty instead of immediately after an activity. When charting is completed near the time that the action was taken, details are much clearer in the mind of the caregiver. Waiting for many hours to chart activities or interactions can produce faulty results in recording nursing care. This is especially true in the larger facilities, where familiarization with individual residents is more difficult. Although this is a preferred method of recording care, exceptions need to be made where unexpected events delay recording of data until late in the day's tour of duty. Anecdotal notes can be written on notepads so long as this information is transferred to the record at the soonest possible time.

Recording Intake of Food and Fluids

Nutritional deficits related to a decrease in appetite or chronic diseases that impair E/LTC residents' ability to chew, bite food, or swallow food and fluids are not uncommon. Assessing these resident care problems and proper recording will trigger a care plan that is specific to the prevention of dehydration and malnutrition. Once triggered, accurate intake must be recorded regularly. The food and fluid intake flow sheets should record the percentage of food and fluids taken at meals, between meals, and for snacks. Charting needs to include any resident care behavior associated with refusal to eat or drink fluids. Dietitian consults need to be recorded, as do any food supplements taken. When family members bring food to their relatives, the type and amount should be recorded on the food and fluid worksheet or on the oral intake record. Notes should be made regarding the name of the person bringing the food and the time that the food is brought into the facility.

Noting a Change in Condition and Follow-Up Care

Keeping the physician of record aware of changes in residents' conditions often is overlooked in E/LTC facilities. When this occurs and the result is that medical attention was not received in a timely manner or was not received at all, litigation is a potential outcome. The term "change in condition" needs to be clearly understood by caregivers. When a resident has a change in condition (improvement or decline), this fact needs to be recorded with the subjective report by the resident or the objective assessment of the caregiver. In the event of an untoward response to a treatment, medication, or plan of care that is in place, a report and recording of specifics are needed. If the assessment is made by nonlicensed caregivers, then the nurse with responsibility for the nonlicensed caregivers must be contacted for further evaluation. All details should be written objectively, clearly, and concisely (Weber and Kelley, 1998). Notification of the physician and family members should be documented with the time of the contact, the family member's name, and the telephone or fax number called. In the event that any of the parties required to be notified is not available, this needs to be recorded, and the follow-up action plan that is to be initiated must be documented.

In most states, injuries or untoward responses that lead to a decline in a resident's condition are to be reported to the Division of Aging. Those states that require notification have specific reporting guidelines. Facilities that care for E/LTC residents need to have a copy of the reporting guidelines available for staff to refer to as needed. In-service education programs that present this information to personnel need to review the content on an annual basis.

When records are examined, the initial change of condition usually is recorded and reported appropriately. The follow-up care is less frequently recorded. When recording a change in condition or the follow-up to a previous change, the nursing assessment must include the recording of vital signs (blood pressure, pulse, respiratory rate, and temperature). The specific change of condition should be named prior to recording the assessment findings (e.g., "Follow-up on fall of 7/4/__"). This type of recording will focus the review on one single event. With record reviews, multiple repeated events of similar character can establish a pattern that will need to be considered in care planning meetings and with the potential for plan of care changes.

Example of a Failure to Report a
Change in Condition and Follow-Up

An example of a follow-up that was not reported but was recorded is the case of a resident who fell in a bathroom. The fall resulted in a 2-inch superficial laceration to the right lower leg, some bruising, but no fractures. The initial reporting and documentation were accurate, and orders were received. A treatment plan for care of the laceration was initiated. It consisted of cleaning the wound and applying a simple nonadhering bandage. The responsible registered nurse did not perform any further assessments but, rather, relied completely on information from the nonlicensed caregivers. Over a period of a week, an inflammation developed, followed by drainage from the cut and then fever. All of these objective findings were recorded but not reported to the licensed nurse. When the elevated temperature was reported to the licensed nurse, a call was made to the physician, and orders were obtained and carried out. Hours later, the resident became septic and then comatose, and death followed within 48 hours.

When the record was reviewed, all objective data were present except for the report to the licensed nurse. Unfortunately for everyone involved, the unreported follow-up problems and the change in the condition of the wound were determined to have contributed to the death. Litigation was avoided when the facility offered an acceptable settlement to the family of the resident.

COMMON AREAS OF
NURSING HOME LITIGATION

Skin Conditions

Skin care programs are in place in all E/LTC facilities. Common skin problems include dry skin, xerosis, skin tears, dermatitis, eczema, herpes zoster, scabies, pediculosis, bullous pemphigoid, skin tumors, and pressure ulcers. The formation of pressure ulcers leads to frequent causes of litigation.

Controversy concerning the preventability of pressure ulcers is ongoing. The Agency for Health Care Policy and Research (1994) published clinical practice guidelines for the treatment of pressure ulcers. These guidelines indicate that "not all pressure ulcers will be prevented, and those that do develop may become chronic" (p. 1).

In the attempt to prevent pressure ulcers, a skin care assessment is completed during the admission process. When individual risks for developing pressure ulcers are identified, a care plan is initiated through the RAP. In the event that a pressure ulcer is present on admission, a treatment plan begins immediately.

TABLE 17.3 Guidelines for Recording Pressure Ulcers

1. Exact location
2. Determine the stage according to Agency for Health Care Policy and Research guidelines: Stage I, II, III, or IV
3. Exact size (including depth)
4. List preventive measures
5. Treatments given
6. Signs of improvement
7. Signs of exacerbation
8. Drainage or odor present
9. Color of tissue in and around pressure ulcer
10. Schedule used for regular treatment and assessment
11. Terminology and methodology must be uniform
12. Physician notification and response
13. Changes in treatments recorded in the medical record and treatment sheets

Follow-up assessments are performed regularly. Some facilities involve physical therapists, nutritional consultants, and skin care specialists to work with the nursing staff to heal a pressure ulcer.

The pressure ulcer assessment includes identifying the exact location of the ulcer and determining the stage and exact size (including depth) of the wound. Preventive measures are fully described. Table 17.3 lists documentation guidelines associated with pressure ulcers.

Skin assessments should be done at least weekly on all residents that are not self-care. If the potential for skin breakdown is known through information obtained on the MDS 2.0 and the RAP, then daily inspections should be done with daily hygiene care.

When a resident is being transferred to another facility or to a hospital for skilled care or surgery, a complete skin assessment is essential. The exception to this is in the case of an emergency transfer. Another complete skin assessment is essential as the resident returns from the other facility or hospital. This recording of the resident's skin condition at the time of leaving and returning to the facility might be important if pressure ulcers or other skin conditions occur while away from the original facility.

Recording the information listed in Table 17.3 in the medical record can provide information related to the assessments, treatments, options for additional treatments, consultations, and (in some facilities) regular photographs of the progress of the ulcer. When litigation ensues due to the formation and/or progression of a pressure ulcer, the jury will be able to follow the care and treatment given with clarity. When the recording is less complete, substandard care can be implied during the discussion of the care and treatment of a pressure

206 DOCUMENTATION IN PRACTICE SETTINGS

TABLE 17.4 Common Causes of Falls

Category A: Extrinsic causes
1. Slipping on floor surfaces
2. Tripping over obstacles in the walk path
3. Misjudging heights of stairs or placement of chairs

Category B: Intrinsic causes
4. Loss of consciousness associated with orthostatic hypotension
5. Drop attacks associated with a sudden loss of muscle tone
6. Seizure-related loss of consciousness
7. Confusion or disorientation, most often associated with falls from beds with side rails in the up position
8. Vertigo that is not associated with a loss of consciousness
9. Pathological fractures that occur prior to the fall

---

ulcer (Lueckenotte, 1996). Little or no information leaves the imagination open to speculate on the outcome.

Falling in the Elderly Population

Falling is one of the most serious and frequent accidents among the elderly population. Falling has been associated with the leading cause of accidental death in persons over 85 years of age. A fall is a symptom of another problem that often results in a more serious problem than the cause that led to the fall. In 1990, the National Institute on Aging estimated that approximately 33% of elderly persons fall in their homes each year. Many fall repeatedly until a serious injury requires medical attention (King and Tinetti, 1995). Table 17.4 lists some common causes of falls.

Five key areas for interventions to prevent falls were identified by Hendrich (1996). The following brief discussion of those key areas provides the basis for implementing a falls prevention program.

The first area is in staff education. Acute care and E/LTC facilities should implement in-service programs that address the risk for falling in the elderly population. Methods for safeguarding the residents from falls must be in place and understood by the staff.

The second key area is in providing assistance and safety during elimination needs. Attempts to reach the bathroom when mobility is impaired and bladder control is weak often cause falls in all settings.

When a risk for falling has been assessed, the resident will need to be monitored for safety in mobility. The third key area is monitoring. The assignment of a one- or two-person assist in walking is important for safety reasons and for continuing to encourage mobility for health reasons. When a determination of a need for one or two persons to assist in walking is made, that decision must be relayed to all nursing staff and placed in a care plan for review by other caregivers.

The fourth key area is environment. A cluttered environment is an invitation to trip and fall. All resident areas need to be assessed regularly for furniture placement, keepsake storage, and cluttered pathways to the bathroom and to the hallway door. In dining rooms, table and chair placement needs to be carefully considered with ease of getting to assigned tables and getting up and down from the chairs at that table. Chairs with legs that are not straight but rather slant outward can result in tripping an unsteady elderly resident.

The fifth and final key area is fall prevention education. Residents, their family members, facility staff, and all caregivers need to be involved in a program of fall prevention. Reminders in areas where falls have been identified as high risk might prove beneficial as an awareness item.

A fall typology with the most common causes of falls was developed by Gray-Miceli (1995). The four areas within this typology are as follows:

1. Multifactorial falls
2. Premonitory falls
3. Prodromal falls
4. Extrinsic falls

Each of these areas is associated with types of physical, mental, or environmental connections with the overall category of falls. Information pertaining to extrinsic falls will provide data that are useful for an environmental checklist in a safety program (Gray-Miceli, 1995).

The reality that falls can occur even with the best education, precautions, and attentiveness to residents must be understood. However, once a fall has taken place, the risk for additional falls becomes much higher. When a history of falls is known, all efforts need to be in place to prevent further falls. Recording the activities taken to prevent falls is essential. When all care is taken to protect residents from falls, those inevitable occurrences will have the documentation needed to separate negligent action from purely accidental events.

The Wandering Resident

The resident who wanders throughout an E/LTC facility should be assessed for the potential of elopement or wandering away from the facility. A confused resident, with a background in physical activity that includes walking, might be at high risk for wandering or elopement. This very difficult management problem occurs with frequency and usually is covered in the media.

Statements often are made by a resident that he or she wants to go home. Attempts to try windows and doors rarely are done in private. Staff members might need to take exceptional efforts to prevent an elopement. Following a first elopement, extreme care must be taken to prevent further attempts to wander away. Exit-seeking behavior is seen as highly motivated and may persist over time (Ebersole and Hess, 1998).

Previous work roles that required walking, lifelong patterns of coping with stress that include walking away from problems, and the search for security somewhere else form three psychosocial patterns of behavior in wandering. During the initial admission interview, information related to these three areas needs to be determined. If dementia is present, then the family will need to make decisions regarding the type of confinement and restrictions necessary to prevent elopement.

Systems for alerting staff of E/LTC facilities when a "wanderer" goes near an exit door have developed over the past decade. These systems include locks that activate in the presence of electronic wrist or ankle bracelets, trunk guards, alarms, and automatic door closures with locks. Electronic tracking devices are being implemented in some facilities for specific needs of persistent wanderers with staunch determination. In the event that the other methods fail, the tracking device will permit a rapid capture and safe return to the facility.

Recording the wandering behavior of a resident and the preventive plan of care is essential when faced with a determined wanderer who is capable of elopement. If a special activity program is initiated such as a facility walking program, then flow sheets or a special activity form should be developed to document this diversional measure to prevent elopement (Holmberg, 1997).

Most claims of negligence occur following an elopement that resulted in the death of the resident. Attorneys involved in these cases will carefully review the thoroughness of the initial assessment, the up-to-date plan of care, and the resident's response to actions to abate wandering and elopement behaviors. These evaluations will look at the involvement of the family in the care planning sessions and the dissemination of the plan of care to all staff members assigned to the areas in which the resident might wander.

Leaving by Choice Versus Elopement

A difference must be established between the resident voluntarily leaving a facility and the cognitively impaired resident who is at risk for harm. When a cognitively oriented resident leaves a facility against medical advice, a report must be made to the physician and family with or without a written statement from the resident. The purpose of leaving should be obtained, if possible. Recording all events that occurred surrounding this situation is of paramount importance. In this situation, the term *elopement* cannot be used and is not considered to be a problem of wandering.

TABLE 17.5 Statements on the Use of Restraints in Long-Term Care

---

The resident has the right to be free from any physical or chemical restraints imposed for purposes of discipline or convenience and not required to treat the resident's medical symptoms. The resident has the right to be free from verbal, sexual, physical, and mental abuse; corporal punishment; and involuntary seclusion.

The facility must develop and implement written policies and procedures that prohibit mistreatment, neglect, and abuse of residents.

The facility must ensure that the resident environment remains as free of accidental hazards as is possible and that each resident receives adequate supervision and assistance devices to prevent accidents.

SOURCE: *Federal Register* (1991, p. 48825).

Using Restraints in Extended and Long-Term Care Facilities

Restraints can be mechanical, physical, or chemical. The use of restraints has decreased over the past decade. Alternatives to restraints are commonly used in most licensed, accredited E/LTC facilities. The switch to alternatives was stimulated by a mandate as stated in the *Federal Register* (1991). This mandate ensures every nursing home resident's right to be restraint free if not required to treat a medical condition (OBRA).

When the use of restraints is done for the protection of the resident or others who might be harmed by the resident, an order must be obtained from the primary care provider. This order can be given after the application of restraints has taken place so long as the behavior that led to the use of restraints is well recorded and follows facility policies. Recording the manner of monitoring the resident throughout the period of restraint and actions taken to reduce the time or use of the restraint is vital. Goals that are set for behavior modification, environmental modification, alternatives considered, and staff involvement in the monitoring process need to be included in the record. Table 17.5 contains the *Federal Register*'s (1991) statement on the use of restraints.

Well-meaning family members often request that restraints be used to prevent falls from wheelchairs and beds when a cognitively impaired resident is agitated and restless. A plan for family teaching should be available for use by the nursing staff that will explain the often increased risk of serious injury when restraints are used for this type of resident. Informing the family of the E/LTC facility's policy on the use of restraints during the admission interview and during care plan meetings is essential to maintain an open line of communication. Changing behavior patterns of confused residents and using alternative actions can reduce or eliminate restraint use (Bryant and Fernald, 1997).

CONCLUSION

LTC has become heavily regulated and, in turn, has fallen prey to litigation. The necessity of accurately completing the MDS 2.0, the RAP, and other forms required by HCFA and OBRA has provided the residents of E/LTC facilities with an in-depth assessment of their unique needs. It is imperative that documentation be completed in the time frames allowed, updated, and reviewed and that plans of care be formulated to satisfy not only the needs of the resident but those of the government agencies as well.

CASE STUDY

Mrs. L, at 86 years of age, was admitted to a nursing home for life care. She often was verbally abusive and combative at home, where her 65-year-old daughter-in-law had attempted to care for her. Mrs. L was diagnosed with multi-infarct dementia not of the Alzheimer's type. The nursing home was a restraint-free facility.

During the first week of residence, Mrs. L entered several other residents' rooms and became verbally abusive with the other residents. She wandered around the dining room yelling that she was a prisoner because her daughter-in-law wanted her money. When staff members attempted to quiet her, she would swing her arms in attempts to hit them. Her behavior was reported to the physician, and orders for a psychological consultation were received.

On the eighth day following admission, she was not found in her room or any other usual place. A search was made of the facility, and she was not found. The local police, the physician, the daughter-in-law, and the Division of Aging were notified in a timely manner. A search within the local area was begun.

Less than a mile away, Mrs. L was found at the scene of an accident, where she had been struck by a car on the neighboring highway. She was pronounced dead at the scene. The driver reported that the woman had stepped out of the shadows and into the lane of traffic. He was unable to stop in time.

The daughter-in-law filed a claim of wrongful death by neglect against the nursing home, on behalf of Mrs. L and her family. The case was settled out of court.

The nursing home owner, administrator, director of nursing, and charge nurse on the unit where Mrs. L resided were named in the litigation. The evidence of failure to protect Mrs. L from harm by elopement was overwhelming. She had verbalized an unhappiness at being in the facility, confusion, and aggressive behavior, and she was very mobile. Although the nursing home was a restraint-free facility, no alarms or locks were placed on exit doors near units with confused residents. No plan of care had been completed for this resident's safety or to manage her behavior problems.

ADVANCED PRACTICE NURSING ISSUES

18

Linda Steele
With Sue E. Meiner

Chapter Outline

The practice of nursing at advanced levels beyond the basic educational preparation has been developing for many decades. However, the term *advanced practice nurse* (APN) does not refer to a singular type of nurse practicing at an advanced level. No standard entry level into advanced nursing practice exists as of 1999.

Clinical nurse specialists (CNSs) with master's degrees have been practicing in many areas of specialization at the advanced level since the 1940s. Nurse practitioners (NPs) have practiced with advanced skills, but not always with advanced educational preparation, since their inception by Loretta Ford in 1965. Certified registered nurse anesthetists (CRNAs) are the oldest advanced nursing specialty. They have only recently been prepared at the master's degree level. Certified nurse midwives (CNMs) traditionally have been educated both in graduate and certificate programs. Nurses without advanced education have been certified as experts in their specialty areas such as critical care nursing (CCRN) by examination and clinical practice.

Because of the multiple educational entries to advanced nursing practice, consumers, other health care professionals, and those within the nursing profession have experienced a great deal of confusion over the roles of advanced nursing practice and the APN. In an effort to clarify the meaning and standardize educational levels of the APN, recent efforts have been made to define the term *advanced practice nurse* and the educational requirements for advanced nursing practice. This chapter discusses current definitions and educational preparation of APNs as well as issues affecting their scope of practice including documentation matters.

DEFINITIONS OF ADVANCED NURSING PRACTICE

Currently, not one accepted definition of advanced nursing practice or of the APN exists. In the American Nurses Association's (ANA, 1995) *Social Policy Statement,* advanced practice refers specifically to advanced clinical practice. This reinforces an earlier position of the ANA (1992) that the four roles encompassing advanced practice are those of the CNS, the NP, the CNM, and the CRNA. Thus, this definition excludes other nurses with advanced degrees such as educators, administrators, and researchers.

Hamric, Spross, and Hanson (1996) differentiated advanced levels of nursing practice from basic levels of nursing by the following characteristics:

1. Specialized in terms of focus and population served
2. Expanded in terms of knowledge and skills
3. Complex in terms of clinical challenges and clinical judgment
4. Independent in terms of decision making (p. 30)

Safriet (1992) defined the APN as

a registered nurse licensed to practice in the state who, because of specialized education and experience, is authorized (certified) to perform acts of prevention, (medical) diagnosis, and the prescription of (medical) therapeutic or corrective measures under regulations adopted by the Board of Nursing. (p. 479)

Advanced nursing practice also is clearly defined in the Nurse Practice Act (NPA) in each state. There is a broad range of differences in these definitions among the various states. Alaska uses Safriet's (1992) definition of an APN. New Mexico takes expanded practice to mean the practice of registered, professional nursing by a registered nurse (RN) who has completed a formal educational program in an institution of higher learning. This person can function beyond the scope of practice of professional registered nursing (New Mexico Statutes Annotated, 1992).

Examples of the definitions of advanced nursing practice in each state can be found in the yearly January issue of *The Nurse Practitioner*. The journal editor compiles a complete directory state by state.

EDUCATION OF ADVANCED PRACTICE NURSES

Although it recently was estimated that two thirds of APNs have been prepared at the certificate level rather than at the graduate level (Mezey and McGivern, 1993), there is now consensus among major nursing organizations and state boards of nursing that graduate preparation is essential for advanced nursing practice. The National Council of State Boards of Nursing (1993) proposed a definition based on licensure as an RN and basic nursing education in addition to a graduate degree with concentration in an advanced nursing practice area. Graduate education is seen as critical in enhancing the credibility of the APN with the public and with other health care professionals (especially physicians).

Autonomy, independence, and increased accountability are inherent in this advanced practice role. Thus, advanced clinical skills, critical thinking, and judgment abilities, as well as a strong theoretical and research base, are essential outcomes of APN graduate education.

CREDENTIALING AND CERTIFICATION

In addition to advanced educational and clinical skills, credentialing by appropriate national professional organizations is required for the APN to practice. The credentialing process leads to national certification in a given specialty area. However, certification is not synonymous with advanced educational preparation, and eligibility requirements to become certified are not uniform at the present time. Each specialty organization determines the requirements. Some nurses without graduate-level education may elect to become certified as experts in their fields of clinical practice, as noted previously. Examples of nationally certified areas of specialization for the APN as NP include adult, family, gerontological, obstetric-gynecology (OB-GYN), and pediatric NPs. Still other examples include psychiatric, cardiovascular, and pulmonary CNSs, CNMs, and CRNAs.

There are many different national organizations that certify APNs. Table 18.1 lists the names of the most commonly recognized certifying organizations for advanced practice in professional nursing.

The American Nurses Credentialing Center (ANCC) has been certifying nurses since 1973, with more than 140,000 certified nurses to date in areas such as CNSs in adult health, adult psychiatric/mental health, community health,

TABLE 18.1 Nationally Recognized Certifying Organizations for Advanced Practice Nurses

- American Academy of Nurse Practitioners
  Capital Station, L.B.J. Building, P.O. Box 12846, Austin, TX 78711
  (512) 442-4262

- American College of Nurse Midwives
  818 Connecticut Avenue Northwest, Suite 900, Washington, DC 20006
  (202) 728-9860

- American Nurses Credentialing Center
  600 Maryland Southwest, Suite 100 West, Washington, DC 20004-2571
  (800) 284-2378

- Council on Certification of Nurse Anesthetists
  222 South Prospect Avenue, Park Ridge, IL 60068-4001
  (847) 692-7050

- National Certification Board of Pediatric Nurse Practitioners and Nurses
  416 Hungerford Drive, Suite 222, Rockville, MD 20850
  (301) 340-8213

- National Certification Corporation for the Obstetric, Gynecologic, and
  Neonatal Nursing Specialties
  P.O. Box 11082, Chicago, IL 60611-0082
  (800) 367-5613

- Oncology Nursing Certification Corporation
  501 Holiday Drive, Pittsburgh, PA 15220-2749
  (412) 921-8597

gerontology, home health, and medical surgical nursing as well as NPs in adult, acute care, family, geriatric, pediatric, and school health.

Other organizations such as the National Certification Corporation for the Obstetric, Gynecologic, and Neonatal Nursing Specialties have more specific practice areas: They certify only OB-GYN/women's and neonatal NPs.

Most organizations require additional education (although not always at the graduate level) as well as advanced clinical preparation with qualified preceptors. The approved candidate may then sit for the certification examination. Once it is successfully completed, the RN is entitled to use the credentials approved by that specialty organization.

DOCUMENTATION FOR RECERTIFICATION

To remain certified, APNs must renew their certification as specified by their certifying body. For example, to renew ANCC certification, the APN must practice 1,500 hours and attend 75 contact hours of continuing education (CE), with options that include publications and teaching formal or CE classes within the specialty

TABLE 18.2 Equivalent Values for Continuing Education Programs

Measurement	Equivalent
1 academic quarter hour	12.5 contact hours
1 academic semester	15 contact hours
1 contact hour	50 minutes
1 contact hour	0.1 CEU (1/10)
1 CEU[a]	10 contact hours
1 CME[b]	60 minutes
1 CME	1.2 contact hours

SOURCE: Adapted from American Nurses Credentialing Center (1997).
a. CEU = continuing education unit.
b. CME = continuing medical education.

over the 5-year period following the original certification date. APNs must maintain meticulous documentation of these credentials to become recertified.

The CE recertification requirements are listed by categories in the ANCC catalog. These categories include specialty area appropriate CE programs that offer either contact hours or CE units. Table 18.2 demonstrates the equivalent measurements of value for CE courses. These can be met with official and unofficial CE offerings. The rule pertaining to the unofficial CE programs is that the content must be applicable to the certification area and usually be presented as an offering in a place of employment. Another source within this category is independent study approved for continuing education units (CEUs) instead of college credit. Items included in this category are home study offerings, CEU programs from publications (journals), and other independent study modules approved by other health professional organizations. An example is a respiratory therapy program for the CNS in critical care management.

The second category is formal education that awards academic credit. The course must apply to the area of certification or be required as part of an advanced degree in the originally certified specialty area. However, general education courses such as history, literature, physical education, music, math, and English do not apply toward acceptable academic credit for recertification.

The third category refers to being a presenter or lecturer to other health care professionals on pertinent topics of expertise. Educators cannot use their full-time work-related class assignments in this category unless they do so as guest lecturers in other relevant courses. Clinical supervision of students can be used to meet some aspects of this category in some specialty certifications.

The final category relates to publishing and research accomplishments for credit toward recertification. Credit for publishing a journal article, a book chapter, or a book that is relevant to the area of specialty is acceptable for up to half of the total recertification needs. The final area within this category is valid if the nurse is one of the recognized researchers in a project that is done during the 5-year certification period.

TABLE 18.3 Recertification Record Keeping

1. Keep all records by the same category as the accrediting agency requires:
   Category I: continuing education credits
   Category II: academic credits
   Category III: presenter/lecturer credits
   Category IV: journal article, book chapter, research project
2. Under each category, highlight the year of completion in bold letters.
3. Maintain the record in a month-by-month order, beginning with the month following your initial certification. When the fifth year has begun, you will have an accurate account of eligible programs.
4. Enter the name of the sponsoring agency or university where the academic credit or the continuing education units were earned. Include the full address and the name of the responsible educational director or registrar whose name appears on the certificate or attendance verification form.
5. List the amount of contact hours, continuing education units, continuing medical education, or credits (quarters or semesters).
6. Keep all original certificates, attendance forms, transcripts, and other accounting materials to submit as proof of fulfillment of the continuing education option for recertification.

SOURCE: Adapted from American Nurses Credentialing Center (1997).

Maintaining these records must be done in a structured manner. Beginning with the first in-service or CEU program following certification, the APN should keep a thorough record of all attendance and CEU points in a hard copy (e.g., written ledger or disk storage) and in a computer-based record system (if available). Table 18.3 provides a suggested format for these records.

THE NURSE PRACTICE ACT AND STATE RULES/REGULATIONS AFFECTING ADVANCED PRACTICE

The authority to practice nursing rests with each individual state and is conferred to the RN through the NPA in that state. Each NPA contains rules and regulations that govern the practice of nursing. The rules and regulations also determine advanced nursing practice in each state. A total of 47 states now have specific provisions in their NPAs controlling advanced nursing practice. These acts define advanced nursing practice and determine the educational and certifying requirements in the state. In Missouri, for example, it is necessary to obtain a certificate of recognition from the state to practice as an APN.

There is a great degree of variability among the states in the interpretation of advanced nursing practice. It is essential that each APN have a copy of the NPA and become familiar with the rules and regulations affecting advanced practice in his or her state. Ignorance of the policies of one's state is no defense in matters affecting advanced practice. These documents can be obtained from each state's Nurse Licensing Board or through the public access of documents from the state's legislative library. This library usually is located in the capital city of the state (e.g., Albany in New York, Jefferson City in Missouri).

SCOPE OF PRACTICE

The scope of practice for the APN is dependent on a variety of factors. Scope of practice is limited by the previous parameters discussed, specifically education, certification, and rules and regulations of various state NPAs. The scope of one's practice can be delimiting, on the one hand, to provide boundaries to frame the depth and breadth of practice. On the other hand, the scope can be broadening to allow for an expanded role with increased expectations and responsibilities. Various issues surrounding scope of practice are examined in the following sections.

CLIENT POPULATION

The type of educational preparation and certification defines the client population approved for APN practice. If the APN graduated from a women's health practitioner program and is certified as such, then she cannot treat men in her scope of practice. For example, if she diagnoses a woman with a sexually transmitted disease, she could not prescribe medication for the partner because that would be beyond her scope of practice. The certified adult NP cannot treat children, nor can the pediatric NP treat adults. Treatment of adolescents is not as clear-cut, so the practitioner's realm of experience and education must be taken into account. The geriatric NP confines patient care to older adults; however, the lower age limit is not clearly defined. The adult NP can care for older persons so long as his or her education, experience, and skills are documented for a random review by the licensing board.

Documentation of education is more easily accomplished with a transcript. Documentation of experience and skills in caring for individuals who might not fit within the stated scope of practice requires a planned and ongoing portfolio. The records should include specific skills that have been learned through observation of an experienced professional practitioner as well as recording the date, location, and initials of the patient when an acceptable return demonstration of the skill is completed. A clinical log or diary is one way in which to keep these records. As the new skill is practiced, the dates, locations, and patient initials should be maintained for review in the event of an audit by the licensing authority.

INDEPENDENCE OF PRACTICE

Autonomy and independence in practice issues are interwoven in scope of practice issues. These concepts are most valued by APNs, and for many, they are the main reason they desired to become APNs. How much autonomy and independence in practice can the APN achieve? Can the APN operate in total independence and hang out his or her own shingle, so to speak? Again, these questions relate directly to scope of practice desired. If the APN wishes to assess, teach/counsel/educate, research, and/or consult, then these actions are within the scope of nursing practice and, therefore, advanced practice. The actions of diagnosis, prescription of medical treatments, and performance of more complex procedures are not totally independent nursing acts in many states. These questions directly relate to the scope of practice of the APN and are addressed both legally and legislatively at the national and state levels.

The answers to these complex questions are found in each state's NPA. As discussed earlier, the license to practice nursing is granted by each state's Board of Nursing, and the advanced practice of nursing also is defined and regulated by most states. Over the past 25 years, state NPAs have evolved to include definitions of advanced practice as well as addressing independent practice. To date, only Alaska and New Mexico allow full independence of practice for the APN. Many states require direct or indirect supervision of the APN by a physician. Some states, such as Missouri, have collaborative practice rules that clearly define the relationship between the APN and the physician (Missouri Nurses Association, 1997; Tadych, 1997). Edmunds (1994) indicated that this type of arrangement is agreeable to physicians because, with the collaborative agreements, the physician retains control over the practice and reimbursement of the APN, and that collaborative practice allows physicians to expand their services to clients as well as reap financial rewards. Areas that are documented within this contract can vary according to the type of practice, location with or without other health care providers, and financial and benefit issues. Chain of command, specified review of records for acceptable practices, and on-call issues need to be clearly written into the agreements (Sebas, 1994).

Safriet (1992), an attorney, recommended that state boards of nursing be empowered to regulate all APN actions without interaction of other regulatory boards such as medicine and pharmacy. Safriet added that statutory requirements for any APN-physician collaborations, practice agreements, supervision, or direction be eliminated.

The collaboration between physicians and APNs may be prescribed by the state NPA and/or desired by APNs. If prescribed by the state, a clear definition

TABLE 18.4 States and Prescriptive Authority for Advanced Practice Nurses

Prescriptive authority (including controlled substances) independent of any required physician authority (17 states): Alaska, Arizona, Colorado, District of Columbia, Delaware, Iowa, Maine, Montana, North Dakota, Nebraska, New Hampshire, New Mexico, Oregon, Vermont, Washington, Wisconsin, and Wyoming

Prescriptive authority (excluding controlled substances) with required physician involvement or delegation (11 states): Alabama, Florida, Hawaii, Idaho, Kentucky, Michigan, Missouri, New Jersey, Nevada, Texas, and Virginia

SOURCE: Adapted from Pearson (1998).

will be found in the rules and regulations of the NPA. For example, in Missouri, the APN is required to have a signed collaborative practice agreement with a physician to be granted prescriptive privileges. This agreement also specifies that the collaborating physician be geographically within a 50-mile radius for APNs practicing in rural areas and within a 30-mile radius for APNs in urban areas (Missouri Statutes, 1995). Appendix A provides examples of collaborative practice agreements.

Prescriptive and Hospital Privileges

The authority to prescribe medications traditionally has been a function reserved only for physicians. Prescriptive authority for APNs is regulated by each state. In 1997, APNs had prescriptive privileges in 47 states. Again, there is great variability. In some states (e.g., New Mexico), the APN has full prescriptive privileges, whereas in others (e.g., Missouri), the APN may prescribe only as delegated by the collaborative practice agreement with a physician. Prescription of controlled substances is allowed in some states as well. Again, the reader is referred to the January issue of *The Nurse Practitioner* for an annual update of prescriptive privileges (Pearson, 1998). Table 18.4 summarizes current prescriptive authority in various states.

ADMITTING PRIVILEGES TO ACUTE CARE SETTINGS

Admitting privileges to acute care facilities or hospitals are granted by each individual institution. Nonphysician providers have been granted hospital privileges since 1983. These privileges are granted to health care providers such as podiatrists, dentists, physician's assistants, and NPs. APNs may apply to hospitals for specific privileges desired such as admitting patients for observation and treatment of health conditions. Consults with physicians can be appropriately made during inpatient stays. Other privileges may be granted at the discretion of the institutional review board according to the education, experience, and skills of the APN.

APNs also may desire to perform specific procedures such as suturing and intubation. Whether or not the performance of specialized procedures is in the scope of practice of APNs is determined by the type of training and experience received. Attainment of some specialized skills such as colposcopy are more clearly prescribed. A formal didactic program is required, as well as a minimum of precepted clinical hours, to become certified to perform this procedure. Other skills such as suturing or endocervical biopsies may be learned on the job or while completing the clinical component of one's educational program. If appropriate training in a specific procedure has not been achieved, then the practitioner should not perform that procedure.

DOCUMENTATION OF PROCEDURES
FOR OBTAINING ADMITTING PRIVILEGES

Documentation of all procedures that have been taught or demonstrated with a return demonstration should be recorded in the APN's portfolio. As opportunities to learn new or improved skills occur, the APN needs to be proactive in learning the procedure. Institutional review boards have the authority to require production of a list of procedures that can be performed based on training and experience. The records maintained by each APN will provide that information if and when it is called on by the subcommittee on privileges. If constraints are placed on the APN, then the value to those accepting care might be too limiting.

STANDARDS OF PRACTICE

Whereas the scope of practice refers to a wide range of factors affecting the practice of the APN, standards of practice are specific measures of behaviors expected of the APN. Standards have been developed to establish minimum levels of acceptable performance and to provide the consumer with a means to measure quality of care. To date, standards of practice for the APN have been developed by national nursing organizations such as the ANA and other specialty organizations. However, the APN must recognize that standards might be too ideal rather than practical because, typically, they are developed by experts and specialists and might not be based on sound scientific research. The APN must have a copy of the standards relating to his or her specialty area and let his or her practice be guided by these standards. In cases of liability, the APN may be judged by these standards.

EMPLOYMENT ISSUES
IN ADVANCED NURSING

There are numerous issues that affect the APN as he or she enters the employment arena to initiate a new role. Discussed here are those surrounding the area of contract negotiation. Most nurses never have experienced the opportunity or necessity of negotiating terms of employment, having worked in institutional settings such as hospitals most of their careers and having accepted carte blanche the terms offered by those institutions such as salary and fringe benefits. Therefore, they are somewhat naive when it comes to negotiating contractual arrangements for employment.

APNs must have a clear understanding of what terms of employment they desire and then be prepared to bargain and negotiate these terms. To develop an understanding of the content, an extensive review of existing contracts is recommended. Many APNs still need to have legal advice in developing contractual agreements. The information obtained in the literature review prepares APNs for the discussions with attorneys. Note that these are separate documents from collaborative practice agreements, as discussed earlier. Negotiating employment terms is an exciting opportunity for APNs to begin a new dimension of advanced practice (Smeltzer, 1991). Appendix A provides a sample employment agreement and a comprehensive employment contract.

CONCLUSION

Advanced practice in nursing is not a new phenomenon. However, there are more nurses entering advanced practice roles than ever before. Although legislative and legal parameters affecting advanced nursing practice are developing at a heightened pace, there are many areas affecting advanced nursing practice in need of clarification. Entry levels into and educational preparation for advanced practice still are not uniform. Credentialing and certification of APNs are performed by many different organizations with varying levels of eligibility requirements. There is variation among the states in definitions and scopes of practice of APNs.

Despite these areas in need of further clarity, the advanced practice of nursing is indeed becoming a critical force in the health care delivery system. APNs have greater opportunities than ever before for becoming health care providers with a broad scope of practice to meet the diverse needs of differing populations of clients. Because of the factors discussed in this chapter, it is important that APNs keep and compile accurate records and documentation affecting the scope of their practice.

CASE STUDY

Sermchief v. Gonzales (1983)

This case directly involved advanced practice nursing in rural Missouri. A group of master's degree-prepared NPs, under affiliation with a physician, conducted a women's health clinic in a medically underserved area of the state. Their care included routine gynecological care with PAP smears, pregnancy testing, and birth control measures, according to written protocols developed by the nurses and a group of supervising physicians. The Missouri State Board of Regulation for the Healing Arts filed suit against the nurses, claiming that they were practicing medicine without a license instead of practicing nursing under the state's NPA.

During the course of this case, briefs detailing the historical development of the nursing profession and the nurse's expanding role in health care delivery were addressed. The Missouri Supreme Court ruled that professional nursing included a broad area of practice and was based on the right to practice nursing within the limits of education and experience. The court held that there was no evidence that the assessments and diagnoses made by the nurses exceeded the limits of their professional knowledge and that the advanced NPs were practicing within the scope of their education and skills and within the scope of nursing as the Missouri legislature had intended.

This case is a prime example of how the nursing profession has and will continue to evolve beyond the traditional nursing roles but within the legal scope of nursing practice. Understanding the various types of nursing practice and having clear knowledge of the legal definitions of the state's NPA are essential. The importance of knowing the content of the NPA in the state where the nurse practices is fundamental to the safety of patients and the legal scope of nursing practice.

NURSING EDUCATORS, ADMINISTRATION, AND NURSING EDUCATION

19

Alice G. Rini

Chapter Outline

Nursing education is a process of guiding changes in attitude, behaviors, and personal philosophy while imparting information about the art and science of caring for humankind, within the performance levels dictated by the legal scope of practice. The unique attributes of the adult learner enrolled in the basic nursing curriculum are both rewarding and challenging to most nursing faculty. This can be due in part to the heterogeneous makeup of the student body in most generic nursing programs. The differing personal values, maturity levels, ages, genders, ethnic backgrounds, and previous life experiences account for the great diversity within nursing programs.

The need to hire educationally and experientially appropriate nursing faculty is paramount to the success of each student. The varied documentation issues that face the professional nurse desiring to enter the field of nursing education are presented in this chapter.

The diverse student body enrolled in basic nursing educational programs has brought about many changes in the manner in which the discipline of nursing is taught. To accommodate all students, learning experiences must be carefully selected to match the needs of each unique student. As students share their individual clinical experiences in pre- and post-conferences, the goal of learning through each other's knowledge is fostered. This is an important step in critical

TABLE 19.1 Academic Personnel Terms

Academic year: This is a period of time during which college and university classes are in session. It usually consisting of two semesters of 15 to 16 weeks or three quarters of 10 to 12 weeks. Summer sessions, intersessions, and winter special sessions generally are not counted in the traditional academic year.

Contract: This is an agreement between two or more parties that creates an obligation to do a specific thing. A contract of employment for faculty, usually in writing, between the employer (the university) and the employee (the faculty) will specify the terms and conditions of employment.

Employment-at-will: This is an employment agreement in which either the employer or the employee may terminate the employment relationship at any time, without notice, and for any or no reason. There are legal and professional limitations on termination.

Tenure: This is status afforded to a teacher or professor on completion of a trial period, thus protecting him or her from summary dismissal. Tenured faculty hold their positions for life or until retirement and may not be discharged except for cause. Titles usually considered in a tenure track are assistant professor, associate professor, and full professor. Lecturers, adjunct faculty, and the rank of instructor are not considered a part of a tenure system.

---

thinking and problem solving that must be learned early in a nursing program in preparation for the more intensive and judgment-based decisions of care that will follow in the final courses.

Documentation of each step of the students' progress is a requirement of many agencies. Some of these agencies are national and regional accreditation organizations, whereas others are professionally based and quite specific to the preparation of the scope of practice. This chapter includes several of the issues that require accurate and timely documentation of the educational process for students and faculty.

ACQUIRING NURSING FACULTY

Faculty in colleges and universities are hired with agreements consistent with typical educational employment, which generally includes a contract for a specific period of time, generally an academic year, semester, or quarter. Schools or departments of nursing adhere to the pattern of the university or college. This differs from typical nursing service or other business and industrial employment, which is generally employment-at-will. College and university employment may include a tenure process (Table 19.1).

There is a formal procedure for documentation in the process of hiring faculty. Some aspects of this process are specific to the academic setting, and some are similar to many other employment settings. In the academic environment, the applicant for a faculty position provides a curriculum vitae to the school of nursing where the professional nurse desires to teach. The curriculum vitae describes the career of the prospective teacher/professor from its beginning, typically from the time of college graduation with the first professional degree to the present. It is a lengthy chronicle, documenting the applicant's education; experience in educational and service settings; scholarship such as grants, publications, presentations, research, and other creative productions; and service activities in employment and community settings. Faculty who are hired must maintain these curricula vitae throughout their careers and typically update their contents on a regular basis. Faculty find that it usually is the best practice to make new entries to their vitae as soon as additions are completed so that the documents always are current (e.g., attendance at a professional conference). Table 19.2 demonstrates a brief sample curriculum vitae.

The faculty search committee, the entity responsible for advertising, interviewing, and hiring faculty and administrators in schools of nursing, has important documentation requirements pursuant to the search process. For each interviewee, the committee maintains a folder with any correspondence, notations on telephone or other contacts, the applicant's curriculum vitae, and the notes and comments from the interview itself. It is recommended that all interviews be conducted in a consistent manner, using an interview schedule comprised of questions to which all applicants will be asked to respond. It is important to note that such a schedule does not have the purpose of stifling a lively and informal discussion with the applicant. It merely ensures that there is a basic consistency across all interviews so that the chance of charges of discriminatory policies being levied is minimized. Search committees usually must report the process and results of the search to university personnel officers, so proper, consistent, and accurate record keeping is imperative.

There are legal requirements that must be observed in the hiring and interview process. Federal laws that influence the hiring process include the following:

Civil Rights Act of 1964. This act prohibits discrimination against a potential employee on the basis of sex, race, color, religion, or national origin in terms of hiring, discharging, or determining salary or other job benefits.

Rehabilitation Act of 1973. This act prohibits discrimination against any qualified handicapped person who would be able, if reasonably accommodated, to perform the job for which he or she applies.

Age Discrimination in Employment Act. This act prohibits discrimination based on age regarding any employment decision for persons age 40 years or older.

Civil Rights Act of 1991. This act extends the earlier laws related to nondiscrimination in employment and provides the opportunity for a jury trial and additional procedural safeguards for applicants and employees.

TABLE 19.2 Sample Curriculum Vitae

Jane R. Doe
55 River Edge Road
Anytown, ST 55555
(707) 555-5555

Education

Bachelor of Science   June, 1980

Major: Nursing; Minor: Philosophy

Honors: Phi Beta Kappa, Sigma Theta Tau

Anytown State University, Anytown, ST 55555

Other university activities: Women's activities editor, 1978-80, *Anytown University Gazette;* women's varsity volleyball, 1977-80 (state championship trophy, 1978); university choir, 1976-80

Master of Science   June, 1983

Major: Primary care nursing practice, adult health; care management

Thesis: Dietary compliance in men with selected cardiac risk factors

Honors: State Nurses Association scholarship, 1982-83; research associate to Dr. Susan Roe, selected through competitive application process

Private University, Sometown, ST 77777

Doctor of Philosophy   May, 1987

Major: Health care ethics and philosophy; qualitative research

Dissertation: Choice of ethical theory in hospital ethics committee decision making

Honors: Who's Who in American Women, 1987; Outstanding Young Women of Anytown, 1987-88

Scholarship

"Use of Ethical Theory by Hospital Ethics Committees," *American Journal of Philosophy,* March, 1989, pp. 67-80

Service

Member, Ethics Committee, Anytown Regional Medical Center, Anytown, ST; term 1994-98

Member, Board of Directors, Anytown Community Center, Anytown, ST; term 1997-99

Professional Activities

Member, Sigma Theta Tau, local chapter, 1980-present

Nominating committee, 1992-93

Scholarship and grants committee, 1997-98

Member, American Nurses Association, 1980-present

Chair, local chapter, 1994-96

State committee, 1995-97

Americans With Disabilities Act. This act prohibits discrimination on the basis of disability if a person can perform the essential job functions. This act adds recovering alcoholics and drug addicts to the category of disabled persons, a provision that has precipitated great controversy, especially in jobs where unimpaired employees are of great importance to the clients seeking their services and where the opportunity for accessing controlled substances is great.

Search committees must document the observance of these laws, typically by completing forms and other records demonstrating compliance. Such records may include a copy of an advertisement confirming the nondiscriminatory nature of the search, the interview schedule, a form revealing the rationale for who is considered/hired and who is not, and minutes of search committee meetings.

That these laws are indeed enforced is demonstrated in several employment decision situations that have been heard in federal court. A recovering nurse drug addict who was restricted from passing narcotics to patients won her case against a hospital that refused to hire her. The court indicated that her addiction was a handicap covered by the Rehabilitation Act and that the refusal to hire her was in violation of the reasonable accommodation rule. This meant that the court required the hospital to hire her to do all nursing duties except administration of narcotics, which someone else would have to perform (*Wallace v. Veterans Administration,* 1988). An appeals court found possible age discrimination in the dismissal of a 62-year-old nurse and remanded the case for trial where hospital administrators commented that "new blood" was needed and that the job was too stressful for the older nurse (*Buckley v. Hospital Corporation of America,* 1985). A pharmacist who was HIV positive was considered not to be a direct threat to patients. The court indicated that his HIV-positive status would not prevent him from accomplishing the job and that the refusal to hire him on the basis of that status was unlawful (*In re Westchester County Medical Center,* 1992). Finally, in *Nassau County, Florida v. Arline* (1987), a teacher with recurring tuberculosis filed a lawsuit when she was discharged from her job because of the disease. The court indicated that any such discharge must be supported by factual and medical evidence to be considered nondiscriminatory.

EVALUATION AND RETENTION OF FACULTY

The contract between the college/university and the professor will specify a period of time, generally 1 academic year, during which there is an employment agreement. This agreement is renewed each year, if approved by a faculty panel and unit administrator, for a series of years, after which the professor may apply for tenure. The annual approval process generally consists of a report by the individual professor to a faculty panel, which might be called a reappointment, promotion, and tenure committee; a personnel and budget committee; a faculty personnel committee; or some similar name. It is comprised of tenured faculty from the School (or Department) of Nursing, usually elected by the nursing faculty group. The function of the committee is to receive the report describing the previous year's activities of the individual (untenured) professor and to evaluate the quality and effectiveness of teaching, scholarship, and service to the college/university and community. These three factors are typical of those evaluated for faculty reappointment. Some colleges/universities also consider collegiality, professional development, and other faculty activities important to the role.

The annual report of each professor is an important document. The report includes items such as new course development, contribution to or preparation of course syllabi, peer evaluations of classroom and clinical practicum teaching, student evaluations of teaching, advisement, grading fairness, respect, and openness to student ideas as well as other activities that relate to the teaching process. In addition to a self-evaluation of the teaching activities, the professor reports scholarly and service activities. After evaluation by the faculty panel or committee, the report is passed on to the unit administrator with a written recommendation with or without reasons for the recommendation, depending on the agreed-on rules of such evaluation. The unit administrator evaluates in a similar manner and then passes on his or her recommendation to a higher level college/university administrator if that is the practice of the particular institution. All the interoffice correspondence and the faculty report are considered permanent documents and are retained and maintained in the faculty file until termination, resignation, or retirement. Table 19.3 provides some academic definitions.

Faculty generally have the opportunity to appeal any of the recommendations from a faculty panel or unit administrator by using the appropriate process. Typically, faculty and administrators are aware of legal and ethical requirements of the evaluation process, and it is likely rare that these processes are in bad faith. If there were evidence of an unfair process (i.e., one that is inconsistent with accepted or contracted process), then an appeal may be heard by a college/university-wide faculty committee or by an independent administrator. Although untenured faculty may experience non-reappointment at the end of a contract period for any reason or for no reason, such non-reappointment may not be due to the exercise of constitutionally protected rights such as speech, press, or religion (*Hillis v. Stephen F. Austin State University,* 1982). Most colleges/universities accept appeals based on process questions only, and substantive decisions belong to the discipline reviewing its own faculty. What this means is that appeals committees do not try to second-guess the school or department in terms of the quality and effectiveness of the activities of the professor as self-reported, only the process by which the decision about reappointment, promotion, or tenure was reached. That process usually is evident in the documentation of the activities and deliberations of the faculty committee, the

TABLE 19.3 Academic Definitions

Teaching: guiding the study of a particular subject; imparting knowledge; instructing through a variety of methods such as precept, example, and experience, with the outcome being the acquisition of knowledge by the learner

Scholarship: the character, quality, activity, or attainments of a scholar; in academia, usually referring to research, study, publication, professional presentation, and grant acquisition that may support the activities

Service: contribution to the advantage of others; in academia, usually referring to committee work, assistance with special projects for the institution, and professionally related activities in the community

Collegiality: formally defined as the relationships among colleagues; in academia, usually referring to mutual support activities, willingness to accept assignments, working well with others, and contributing positively to the department or school

Professional development: activities, continued learning, and special practice that expand the professor's technical, intellectual, and/or ethical standards

administrators, and the report of faculty activities. Therefore, contemporaneous recording in the form of minutes is of the utmost importance. In support of college/university decision making, in *Batra v. Board of Regents of University of Nebraska* (1996), the court stated that there is no denial of procedural due process for an untenured faculty member who is not reappointed to a faculty position because there is no interference with a property right.

After a specific number of years of academic employment, a professor may apply for tenure and/or promotion to a higher professorial rank. Faculty are hired as instructors, assistant professors, or associate professors, depending on the hiring agreements at the institution. Annual contracts are awarded (as described earlier) to those faculty recommended for reappointment until a final year, usually the sixth or seventh year, when the instructor or assistant/associate professor *must* apply for tenure or resign from his or her position. During the years preceding tenure, the individual is expected to be highly productive with expanding and increasing scholarly and service activities as well as continuous improvement in teaching effectiveness, all measured by the standards of the particular college/university. Although these activities are documented each year in the faculty annual report, in the tenure year, the faculty member must prepare an extensive application that describes activities and accomplishments in the areas required by the college/university during the entire pre-tenure period. Applications for promotion are similar to those for tenure and are expected to consider several years of work. It can be said that the documentation of a professorial career is never-ending and is one of the more important record-keeping activities of the role.

Schools and departments of nursing have individual characteristics, as do colleges and universities. The former tend to follow the patterns of the latter.

Such characteristics determine whether the pre-tenure years are supportive to developing faculty or are competitive for them. In some institutions, faculty are nurtured through the reappointment and tenure process. Senior faculty provide opportunities for junior faculty to participate in grants and to contribute to publications, and they recommend junior faculty for committee memberships and special projects. In other institutions, however, the process is highly competitive, and junior faculty must find their own opportunities or fail to be reappointed in any pre-tenure year or be denied tenure in the final year. Other differences include where the emphasis is in terms of faculty activities—teaching, scholarship, or some other single activity or mix of activities. Faculty are well advised to clearly document their activities, particularly in the area(s) demanded or favored by the institutional process.

DISCIPLINARY AND GRIEVANCE POLICIES AND PROCEDURES

Part of the contract with a college/university includes a process for disciplining incompetent faculty and those who act improperly. Much as other industries have an escalating discipline process, colleges/universities also provide a means to identify problems with a faculty member and either ameliorate them or terminate his or her position. The issues unique to the academic setting are the contract and the tenure system. Because tenure confers a property right to the faculty position, the process for threatening that right generally is more extensive and requires more processes. After tenure is conferred, a faculty member may not be discharged, except for cause, without due process (*State ex rel Keeney v. Ayres*, 1939; *State ex rel Richardson v. Board of Regents*, 1953; *Zumwalt v. Trustees of California State Colleges*, 1973). In addition, at least one court has determined that findings of college/university panels may be reviewed by courts to determine whether the cause for removal was supported by the evidence (*Zumwalt*). This points up the importance of documentation of problems and general evaluation of faculty. If faculty dismissal for cause is contemplated, then the college/university decision must be free of evidentiary problems due to potential court challenges to this type of dismissal. For probationary faculty or those not yet tenured, the disciplinary process deals only with the contract period. Policies and procedures generally are reduced to writing in a faculty handbook, which serves as the contract provisions governing the faculty-institution relationship. Most colleges/universities provide for a faculty-driven process that includes peer evaluation during the annual reappointment process (described earlier) as well as review of faculty with competence or other problems. Faculty are subject to the same problems as are employees in other industries—incompetence, impairment due to alcohol or drugs, improper acts such as excessively personal or sexual relationships with students, and failure to meet job requirements.

Documentation in the disciplinary process is formal and extensive. When a problem is identified, the professor is asked to attend a meeting to discuss the concerns, and a letter is placed in the permanent record. If the problem continues, then a written notice of the deficiency is given to the professor by the appropriate administrator. The notification often is accompanied by documentation of the deficiency. The professor then has the opportunity to refute or rebut the evidence of the deficiency. This process may occur in the nursing academic unit exclusively or may include the deliberations of a college/university-wide committee or panel of peer faculty, generally all tenured, to review the documents that support and contradict the deficiencies or problems alleged. Recommendations from the nursing unit or the faculty committee generally go to the chief academic officer of the college/university, who has the final decision-making authority regarding the professor's retention or termination. This is all part of due process, which is a constitutional protection in the Fifth and Fourteenth Amendments to the U.S. Constitution and in most state constitutions. *Black's Law Dictionary* describes due process of law as requiring a competent tribunal, which in the public courts means one appropriate for the subject matter of the case (Black, 1991). In the college/university, such a tribunal is described in the faculty handbook and in the contract of employment accepted by the hired professor, and the decisions of this tribunal are valid if the essential elements of due process are followed in the disciplinary process.

Due process is an orderly proceeding in which a person is served with notice of a problem and is afforded the opportunity to be heard and to protect his or her rights before an organizational body having the power to hear and decide such cases (Black, 1991). Often, the contract salary must be paid even if the professor does not return to the classroom, unless there are extraordinary circumstances. Documentation of this disciplinary process includes the original allegation with evidence and appropriate exhibits; the professor's rebuttal with evidence or explanation, other testimony from peers and/or students, and exhibits as needed; the response and record of the deliberations of the administrator and/or committee with a letter of recommendation for solution to the academic officer and the professor; and, finally, the decision and correspondence from the chief academic officer to all of the parties. This documentation is retained by the college/university in case it needs to defend its position in a civil court. Because the loss of a faculty position or even significant discipline within it might damage the professor's academic and personal reputation, careful documentation and compilation of evidence is of the utmost importance. Such loss or damage to reputation that is not well founded is open to redress in civil court under a theory of defamation. Unlike the non-reappointment decisions that merely avoid renewing a lapsing contract for an additional year, discipline for deficiency or wrongful acts might more readily find its way into the courts where the collegial atmosphere and peer involvement do not exist. In fact, in *Zumwalt*, the court indicated that even where there is no property right threatened such as tenure, where there is the possibility of damage to reputation, a hearing might be needed. As stated previously, although courts generally do not involve themselves in substantive academic decisions about the quality of teaching and scholarship, where reputations are at risk, the tort of defamation is an issue that may well be litigated. Where material facts are in question, a hearing also might be needed if such facts would have a deleterious effect on reputation (*Yucker v. University of Florida*, 1992). A well-documented and good-faith process will forestall problems or reversals for the college/university in court.

One documentation issue that is problematic is that of confidential file material that is maintained after an investigation of sexual harassment in the workplace. Employers are correctly investigating all complaints of such harassment thoroughly to avoid having legal problems with the sexual harassment laws. If the complaint was justified, then corrective action would likely be taken and documented in the harasser's file. But if the complaint was not justified, perhaps the result of some conflict, bad faith, or misunderstanding, then there is some concern as to how to document the complaint and its subsequent investigation. If there is no record kept, then if there is a subsequent complaint, there is no record of a possible pattern. If the record is kept, then it is possible that an unfounded accusation might remain in an employee's personnel file or at least in someone's file, perhaps in the human resources department. It is conceivable that such information could be improperly revealed at some time in the future. Employees should be familiar with the organizational policies about record keeping concerning complaints or problems so that they can protect themselves from negative information that might have been remedied long ago or might be incorrect.

CONFIDENTIALITY OF STUDENT RECORDS AND GRADES

Nurses are keenly aware of the need for confidentiality of client/patient records, and the need for similar care exists in the schools. The law controlling student records in postsecondary schools is the Family Educational Rights and Privacy Act of 1974 and the Buckley Amendment to that act. At the time of the passage of this act, few states had laws protecting the release of student information to others and providing for access to those records by students and their parents. The act's provisions included any school, public or private, receiving federal funding from any program administered by the U.S. Department of Education. The Buckley Amendment specifically provided for the students' rights to access their school records, to have information about how to attain such access, and to consent to the release of those records to persons other than faculty and other institutional personnel with a legitimate educational interest in the information or pursuant to a court order for release. Also in the act were provisions for students to challenge information to which they might object (Brent, 1997). Other issues addressed by the act included that students may not review letters of recommendation if they have signed releases with regard to them and that students who wish to be notified of receipt of letters of recommendation be so notified. Parents do not have access to records of medical or psychological treatment, and students do not have access to personal notes made solely for the use of the teacher or administrator who makes them (Brent, 1997).

Student grades are important records maintained by the college/university. There is a formal process for the notification of students about final course grades in a particular quarter or semester. Faculty provide grade lists to the registrar of the college/university, who then generally sends them by mail in the form of transcripts or grade reports. Grades usually go directly to the students, unlike in the past, when the grades of students under 18 years of age went to their parents or guardians. The students then have permanent written records of their grades for each semester. They also may obtain cumulative reports that list all grades earned for all semesters/quarters during which they were in attendance at the particular institution. One of the issues that has been of concern to faculty and students is the notification of interim grades such as those from examinations and other assignments for which students do not receive some document returned from the faculty with comments and a grade. Those grades often have been posted on bulletin boards or in some other areas. Attempts have been made to reduce the likelihood that grades would be revealed to persons with no right to that information. The use of social security numbers was popular for a time, but because such numbers often are listed alphabetically on a class list, it was not difficult for other persons to determine who received what grades. Furthermore, even with nonalphabetized numbers, the first three digits of the social security number can reveal a person's geographic origin, at least the location in the country where the number was issued. This might cause grade information to be divulged improperly. Some schools assign arbitrary numbers that only the students know. Some faculty evaluate students' work using only numbers rather than students' names. Faculty generally have adopted some notification process that preserves students' privacy while timely informing students of their grades.

DUTY TO CARE FOR PATIENTS OF NURSING STUDENTS

Nursing faculty have a unique position in the health care system. They usually are not employed by the health care institution in which they supervise students, yet they often have responsibility for a group of patients for whom those students provide nursing care in a clinical practice situation. Schools and departments of nursing have contracts with the health care facilities in which the students practice, and those contracts always are expected to be in writing. They document the agreements between the schools and the health care agencies. Contracts typically address who is responsible for clients/patients, what privileges are available to students and faculty, and what consideration is expected for the privileges. Although there rarely is an exchange of money between institutions, there has been some emerging expectation of such an arrangement.

Expectations of health care agencies include the requirement of faculty competence in the particular clinical setting. Students generally are not considered in the staff count, so the presence of students does not affect the number of staff assigned to work for the particular unit or shift. Staff nurses assigned to clients/patients for whom students are providing care generally retain responsibility for those clients/patients. However, faculty supervising students and maintaining contact with those patients have the responsibility to make appropriate assessments and report findings that might require the intervention of the staff nurse. Competent faculty supervising prepared students are actually a benefit to an agency unit or function because they provide additional observation of the clients and often special, more individualized care given that each student often has only that one client for whom to care. Documentation of such care by the student is expected to be consistent with agency policy and to conform to all documentation and charting standards required by that particular agency or agency type.

NURSING EDUCATION ADMINISTRATION

Prelicensure programs of nursing must be approved by state authority and generally seek accreditation by a professional association recognized for its accreditation activities. The accreditation organization most recognized is the National League for Nursing (NLN) based in New York. The NLN accredits nursing programs at all levels—practical nursing, associate degree nursing, diploma nursing, baccalaureate nursing, and graduate programs leading to the master's and doctoral degrees. The accreditation criteria are developed by the NLN with the collaboration of its member schools and are published for the edification of the member schools. When schools seek accreditation by the NLN, which is a voluntary process conferring some recognition of excellence, they must respond to each published criterion in terms of how they fulfill it and supply independent evidence of such compliance. The criteria are general in nature and address the operations and outcomes of the educational process. The self-study or report to the NLN by a school seeking accreditation is a lengthy and substantive document reviewing all the curricular activities, personnel, resources, and student information for a period of years.

STUDENT DISCIPLINE AND DISMISSAL

Academic Standards and Grading

Nursing education in the college/university is similar to education in other disciplines and majors. Grading methods must adhere to the institution's stated policies. Standards for demonstrating mastery of content cannot differ significantly from such standards in other departments and schools within the college/university. There are, however, some unique issues in grading and content mastery in nursing. Nursing education shares characteristics with many of the practice disciplines that may be found in higher education such as teaching, social work, and performing arts. Grading is not simply a measure of what students achieve on examinations, written papers, and oral presentations.

To be sure, nursing students must perform adequately in these objective or in-classroom assignments. It is not difficult for a student to be dismissed from nursing school because of failure to achieve a passing standard in the classroom. There could, of course, be a claim that an assignment did not actually test pursuant to the course objectives or that a test or assignment was unfair. Generally, if all students were subject to the same assignments graded by the same criteria, then such claims would be dismissed, although some issues of evenhandedness when grading papers or presentations might have some merit. To avoid such claims, nursing schools strive for internal consistency in their curricula and grading. This means that a course description and learning objectives are presented in writing to students in the form of a course syllabus and that assignments and the grading thereof are closely related to the learning expected in the course. If there are subobjectives for each educational unit within a course, then those also are in the syllabus or a longer document, the course outline. Students know all of these elements in the beginning of the course, although in some cases, additional content might be added with adequate notice to students. Nevertheless, subobjectives must relate to the major course objectives, and testing and grading of such subobjectives must be consistent with stated learning expectations. Assignments and criteria for evaluation should be included in the syllabus. Faculty may also grade written and oral work using a grading form that enumerates the grading criteria and provides a grade and comments relating to the student's performance for each criterion. Such specificity in grading makes it clear to the student, prior to completing the assignment, what will be graded and how much of the grade is for substance or content and how much is for form, such as writing quality and references. Such documentation is helpful to the faculty in defending a grade if the need were to arise and to the student in determining where the best work was done or not done. It also is helpful in creating a permanent record of the student's work and his or her grade if the nursing administrator were to need to explain or defend faculty action to an accrediting body or a complainant. Passing or failing grades in such a system are clear, and academic failure and dismissal for such failure is straightforward. It is interesting to note that at least one court was of the opinion that a student was denied due process when terminated for poor scholarship without a hearing (*Ross v. Pennsylvania State University,* 1978). The court indicated that a hearing was a minimal burden to the university and that such a process would have afforded the student an opportunity to explain mitigating circumstances. This court did not overturn the dismissal; rather, it only required additional process, after which the same decision might be made.

Schools generally have policies that indicate how many times courses may be repeated after a failure. When the student runs out of retakes, he or she will not be readmitted to the nursing school or any of its courses. It is, of course, important that schools adhere to their policies for all students so that no claim of inconsistency or discrimination will hold against the school when any dismissal occurs. Some courts have addressed the student grading issue. In *McIntosh v. Borough of Manhattan Community College* (1980), a student failed a course in the second and final opportunity by 0.287 points. The court stated that it would not interfere with the administrative discretion of faculty and college unless it could be shown that the discretion was improper and that there was no need to justify not rounding the grade to the next highest point for the student to pass the course given that the college had no policy to support such action.

Electronic Media for Course Material

An interesting publication process for course syllabi and outlines is emerging in this electronic age. Whereas in the past such documents were published on hard copy (paper), it is now common to publish them electronically on the Internet. Of course, the same standards apply; faculty must provide syllabi and outlines to students, and students are responsible for the content and provisions within them. Instead of receiving syllabi on the first day of class, students may have access to such documents well prior to that time merely by going to the homepage or World Wide Web site of the college/university, the academic department, or the professor to find the documentation needed. Notifications of changes made by the professor can be automatically communicated to students via e-mail. Notification of e-mail from a professor can be either in a startup message if so configured in the student's computer or by accessing one's e-mail provider. All parties involved have documentation of the sending and receiving of the change message because the professor will be notified of the successful receipt of messages by students or an error message that some e-mail sent did not arrive at a particular destination. It is almost better than contemporaneous documentation in a calendar or planner of such action by a professor because it is done automatically and is retained in the professor's computer until deleted. The electronic age has made documentation of action much more convenient and foolproof.

Disciplinary Dismissal

Dismissal from nursing school for actions other than academic failure is not as clear or straightforward a process. There are additional expectations of students when dealing with external health care agencies and patients in terms of ethical behavior, maintaining confidentiality, and ensuring patient physical and psychological safety. It is not always possible to clearly delineate these because every breach of ethics, confidentiality, and safety cannot be enumerated in a syllabus before the fact. An inadvertent act without malice that does little or no damage might serve as a single element in a pattern of behavior yet to be observed, which is documented and discussed with the student but not cause for immediate dismissal from a nursing program. Another act might be so grievous that it requires immediate expulsion. These dismissals are difficult for the school, the faculty, and the student. Actions that are problematic yet not specifically predictable pose an issue of notification. If there is not documentation of all expected standards, then students can claim that they were not aware of such requirements. On the other hand, it can be reasonably demanded that certain behaviors are inherent in the nursing role and that such generalizations provided in syllabi could be construed to include prudent judgment by even beginning nursing students. Decisions about evaluation and grading are the responsibility of the faculty, but they must not be made capriciously, arbitrarily, or in a discriminatory manner (Brent, 1997). Courts have ruled that faculty decisions about student evaluations are within the academic realm only and that they will not intervene because courts are not equipped with the academic expertise to make such determinations (*Board of Curators of the University of Missouri v. Horowitz,* 1978).

The clearer and more frequent the notice of deficiency to the student, the better the faculty is in compliance with due process obligations due the student (Brent, 1997). Courts have given great respect to the professional judgment of faculty and have stated that they will not override such decisions unless they are a substantial departure from accepted academic norms (*Regents of the University of Michigan v. Ewing,* 1985). In terms of notice, one court indicated that procedural due process was satisfied if a student had prior notice of unsatisfactory performance and the possibility of dismissal. The court further stated that the dismissal decision must be careful and deliberate (*Schuler v. University of Minnesota,* 1986). Such pronouncements make clear the absolute need for ongoing, detailed documentation of student performance, particularly of clinical or similar activities. It also is wise to institute regular recording of student performance rather than just documenting errors or problems because the latter could be construed as one-sided or harassing.

Anecdotal Notes

Faculty are advised to document carefully the problems that a student might have that could precipitate dismissal. Anecdotal notes kept by the faculty and written notice to the student are minimum requirements. Personal anecdotal notes used by the clinical professor exclusively generally are not discoverable and will not likely be required as evidence in court. Notes entered into official student records are, however, discoverable. Faculty are advised to make only objective, impartial, and unbiased statements in official student records.

Whereas many faculty members use anecdotal notes to maintain a detailed accounting of poor student performance, other teachers keep anecdotal notes on all outstanding student experiences and performances. The most common use of student-based anecdotal notes is with a clinical group. Using the class list and a comments area for brief narrative remarks, the instructor can describe positive events and areas that need improvement. If the anecdotal notes are kept as documentation for clinical evaluations, then they become a part of the student's file and are discoverable.

STUDENT LIABILITY FOR PATIENT CARE

Nursing students are personally liable for their own wrongs and negligent acts. Even nursing students under the age of majority are not exempt from the responsibility to act in a reasonably prudent manner while caring for assigned patients (Hershey, 1965). The standard of care expected by any patient is not lowered due to being cared for by a student nurse. To ensure the safety of patients while protecting themselves from liability claims, student nurses must be prepared to care for assigned patients. The student nurse must be able to recognize skill limitations and seek assistance from the instructor or other registered nurses if the student nurse realizes that he or she is inadequately prepared to render safe nursing care.

Clinical experience is obtained by the educational institution, from health care facilities, through a contract. The standard and usual contract requires that the nursing program send only those students whose health and academic progress meet the test of an ordinary, reasonable, and prudent nursing student in a clinical experience situation. The health care agency agrees to accept a specific number of students and instructors on predetermined nursing care units for prescribed times and dates (Trandel-Korenchuk and Trandel-Korenchuk, 1997).

A state of Virginia court held the opinion that it is not sufficient to say that a nurse is competent simply because he or she is capable of discharging the manual duties incumbent on him or her as a nurse. If the nurse is lacking in educational preparation, if he or she is guilty of indiscretion that impairs her physical or mental status, and if he or she is lacking in that moral character that imbues the patient with confidence, then it cannot be said that the nurse is a competent person to be placed in charge of a helpless patient (*Norfolk Protestant Hospital v. Plunket,* 1934).

Documentation of successful performance of nursing skills can be initiated by the first clinical instructor in the program. The documentation record should grow with every clinical experience until all skills, contained within the legal scope of practice, are performed at an acceptable level. The documentation can be in the form of a checklist of skills. An advantage of the checklist is that it can be made available to the nurse manager on the assigned unit. When this is done ahead of time, the assignment of staff nurses can be made to enhance the skill levels of the students preparing to receive clinical practice.

PLAGIARISM

Student writing and other performance is expected to be the work of that student, and if outside sources are used to produce the student's work, then those sources are to be cited according to some designated and appropriate format. The American Psychological Association format is well accepted in academic organization, as are the formats of the American Sociological Association, Harvard Blue Book, MLA, and others. The purpose of citation is to give credit to the original author for the ideas, the information, and the research and to assist the reader in locating the original source. Plagiarism is the act of appropriating the ideas, words, or language of another and passing them off as one's own (Black, 1991). Plagiarism usually is grounds for failure on the work in which the plagiarism is found, but in some colleges/universities, it is grounds for course failure and dismissal from the school. Students are well advised to learn the documentation and citation process and to use it consistently in all the work they do. Faculty, too, must be knowledgeable about citation in all that they write or present.

CONCLUSION

Documentation is a fact of life in academia. There are formal requirements in documenting all dealings with faculty, from the recruitment and hiring process through the evaluation, promotion, and dismissal processes. Proper and timely documentation helps avoid any procedural difficulties in these processes. Faculty themselves are bound to accurate and appropriate documentation of their own endeavors and of their evaluation and record keeping related to student activities. The documentation related to student evaluation, grades, and clinical functioning is complex and essential for the accreditation, state approval, and proper functioning of the school. Knowledge of the law as it relates to university-professor and faculty-student relationships will direct what documentation is needed and advisable in most situations.

CASE STUDY

Atkinson v. Traetta (1974)

In this case, all the students in a nursing program were informed in the process of their nursing education that a D grade no longer would be acceptable in any nursing course and that for a student to progress in the program, a C grade or better was needed. Anything less than a C would require repeating the course pursuant to school policy regarding repeats. (It is worth noting that many nursing schools permit only one repeat; that is, a course may be taken only two times, and only a limited number of courses may be repeated in any program.)

Because of the change in grading standards, several students were unable to progress in the nursing program. When these students enrolled in the program, the passing grade was D. It was during their continued enrollment that the change was made. The students filed a suit asking for an injunction allowing them to continue in the program. They claimed that the change amounted to a curriculum change that occurred after they had enrolled and, therefore, violated their contractual agreements with the college as described in catalog curricular requirements. The college/university catalog is considered the contract between the student and the school. If curricular changes are made, then students already enrolled usually are not required to meet the new requirements but, rather, are held to the requirements in effect at their time of enrollment in a program.

In *Atkinson*, the trial court found for the students and granted the injunction. The faculty, however, asserted that the change constituted a grading change that addressed the need for demanding high standards for passing nursing courses. They insisted that it was not a curricular change given that no course requirements were changed. On appeal, the New York State Appellate Division Court reversed the trial court decision and held that the change that required students to achieve a C grade or better was not a curricular change but, rather, definitely a grading change. The court further held that even if it was a curricular change, the faculty were acting to uphold high academic standards, and such standards were particularly important considering the clinical component of the courses and the public's safety. The court also noted that the grading change was communicated to the students well in advance of the effective date of the change, giving students time to adjust their notions of what constituted a passing grade.

MANAGED CARE　20

Sue E. Meiner

Chapter Outline

Traditional health insurance, called indemnity insurance, and fee-for-service payments have been the mainstay of paying for health care services until economic conditions caused a need for better financial management of the health care dollar. In a move to curb the serious escalation of national health care costs, a system called Managed Care (MC) evolved (Trandel-Korenchuk and Trandel-Korenchuk, 1997). The dynamic development of MC has taken several different directions. These differing concepts of what MC is and is not have created confusion among health care providers and patients.

ENVIRONMENTAL CHANGES IN HEALTH CARE DELIVERY

The pressures to contain health care costs have forced health care providers to change the styles of health care delivery. The hospital component is experiencing enormous adjustments to this change in focus. Patients are admitted for treatment in the later stages of diseases, surgical stays can be a few hours after a procedure to a single day or less (23-hour admissions). According to McCloskey and Grace (1990), "Their treatment involves a high level of technological care that requires counterbalancing by 'high touch' on the part of nursing staff" (p. 166).

TABLE 20.1 Managed Care Organizations

Payer-based organizations: Costs of services are provided under health plans that are paid for by individuals or sponsoring companies. Examples of these organizations include the following:

- Indemnity insurance companies: These supply services according to a benefit plan that is paid by the individual or employer as a premium charge.
- Blue Cross/Blue Shield Groups: Health care services are paid through agreement with providers of care, usually at a discounted rate.
- Health maintenance organizations: These are prepaid health care plans that combine the payment plan and the health care services. The staff model is used when physicians and nurse practitioners are employees of the system for contracted salaries.
- Self-insured plans: The organization is large enough to be able to collect premiums or contribute the costs of services through establishing reserve funds sufficient to cover anticipated health care costs. These plans are monitored by most states through government insurance agency oversight offices.

SOURCE: Adapted from Johnson and Niederman (1996).

Managed Care Structures

Among the variety of MC structures are the independent practice association (IPA) and the preferred provider organization. The oldest of managed care organizations (MCOs) is the health maintenance organization. Although MC has not developed uniformly into a single system, the premise is to provide the patient with appropriate care given by an appropriate health care provider for the level of care needed. The coordinating of all health care services is central to the philosophy of MCO (Trandel-Korenchuk and Trandel-Korenchuk, 1997). Table 20.1 lists some of the different MCOs.

Currently, the three types just named have grown into many varieties including mixtures of two or more of the original types. Utilization management companies have expanded into providing services for other types of MCOs, further confusing the overall understanding of the MCO system.

Medically Necessary Treatment

Of concern to the general public and health care providers is the matter of limitations in payment of services based on a schedule of fixed payments for specified services, regardless of the individual nature of a patient's needs. The requirement for preapproval for services, other than clearly identified emergency care, has led some patients to obtain services that were not paid by the MCO, causing personal financial stress. Some health care services might not be covered by some MCOs but are covered by other MCOs. Each MCO establishes guidelines for patient care, referral, and reimbursement. In most cases, little selection of a primary health care provider or hospital is available. In larger health care service environments, a larger selection of centers and providers is afforded to the subscribers of the MCO. The courts in several states have reprimanded some MCOs for denial of medical care reimbursement or preapproval of services based on unreasonable decisions for the denial of payment (Trandel-Korenchuk and Trandel-Korenchuk, 1997).

La Puma and Schiedermayer (1996) stated, "Defined contractually, and sometimes retrospectively, it [health care service] is an administrative judgment based on contractual language. It may not coincide with an individual practitioner's clinical judgment" (p. 93).

UTILIZATION REVIEW VERSUS
QUALITY IMPROVEMENT PROGRAMS

When MCOs initiate their own or contract with an independent third party for utilization review/management services, the focus is on cost-effective delivery of health care. According to Johnson and Niederman (1996), "Utilization review and management programs are designed to [en]sure that only medically necessary services are provided and that services are provided in a cost-effective manner consistent with good clinical outcomes" (p. 15).

Quality improvement (QI) programs direct attention to the promotion of the delivery of care within standards of care while monitoring the clinical outcomes of services provided to subscribers. When deficiencies are identified, corrective actions are taken to provide education and assist in the change process to eliminate the deficiencies. Areas initially identified are then monitored for continuous quality of service and for determining the long-term effect of the change.

QI programs begin with patient services. Because nursing care provides the basis for hospital care, the QI program begins with collecting data related to a specific problem that is or has been identified by a member of the health care team. The standard areas to review for these concerns are those that are labeled as high risk, high volume, or high cost.

An example of high risk is in the care of indigent pregnant teenagers admitted to a public hospital for delivery without prenatal care. High volume in this case might be the same identifier (patient profile). High cost might be the length of stay of this identifier due to complications associated with a lack of prenatal care. Data are collected on each of these areas and are analyzed. The solution or corrective measures might include a free, nonjudgmental maternity clinic in economically disadvantaged neighborhood locations. The costs of this clinic might offset the costs of critical care obstetric services in the hospital for both mother and baby. The outcome measures might be a healthy experience for mother and baby as well as savings to the community for very expensive neonatal care for the baby.

JOB ROLE STANDARDS OF PERFORMANCE

New liability concerns have emerged in connection with MC. One such concern relates to the multiple role functions of a single individual within an MCO. In small offices, one licensed nurse can be responsible for all office functions, admission assessments, pharmacy contacts, patient teaching, and telephone triage without direct supervision of a primary care provider. Regardless of the roles, all actions must meet the standards of performance according to policies and procedures including, but not limited to, the job description (Johnson and Niederman, 1996).

Ethics and Business Conflicts

Although ethical decision making is a constant issue in the health care settings, some ethical issues are more business related than bioethical. An example of this issue is in the case of a health care provider—nurse practitioner (NP), part-time contractual services with two MCOs—who must bill for services in one MCO at a significantly lower fee, and with abbreviated services, than in a different MCO, for which a higher rate and expanded services are permitted.

Although the same standards of care are required, the disclosure of the plan with improved services cannot be discussed with the patient as a provision of the contract for services. Disclosure could be identified as a conflict of business interest if a patient were to switch to another plan based on the discussion of services (Johnson and Niederman, 1996).

ROLE OF THE ADVANCED PRACTICE NURSE

MCOs retain physicians as the primary gatekeepers of health care for subscribers to their services. Negotiations for advanced practice nurses (APNs) to share in primary care of patients currently are under way. In some areas of the United States, negotiations have been successfully completed, and APNs are in primary care practice with physicians in MC (Guido, 1997).

The cost-effectiveness of the MCO industry has led to studies comparing the savings of physician-only primary practices to those of physician and NP practices. Appleby (1995a, 1995b) found that practice revenues demonstrated that primary care practices with physicians and NPs cost 40% less than did physician-only practices. This cost-effectiveness was due in large part to the NPs' multidimensional expertise in counseling, health teaching, and case management.

According to the American Academy of Nurse Practitioners (1997), "A combination of health care providers including physicians and NPs [is] needed to address the cost-effective and care-effective challenges of comprehensive health care with a personal caring focus" (p. 1).

CREDENTIALING AND PRIVILEGING PROCESS IN THE MANAGED CARE ORGANIZATION

The process of verification of the NP's education, skills, and experience to provide primary health care to patients is termed *credentialing*. Traditional information required for nurse credentialing involves the basic verification of education (nursing program graduation), licensure, advanced degrees, and certifications. Additional areas involve professional organization memberships, offices held in these organizations, teaching experience (and references from former instructors), and any history of liability issues. Rustia and Bartek (1997) defined this issue as follows: "Credentialing is the process by which the professional provides evidence [that] he or she is qualified to perform designated clinical activities" (p. 90).

Credentialing for physicians is more complicated in that it involves information related to performance measures, financial disclosures related to hours of availability throughout the day and week, and accessibility to patients. Other matters include physical and mental health status and the history of all previous practices (work settings).

The privileging process pertains to peer review of professional skills, work attitudes, and competence. This is the area that requires the maintenance of records related to all continuing education, practice experience, and skill in performing specific procedures. Rustia and Bartek (1997) defined this process as follows: "Privileging is the process through which the employing organization grants a professional specific authority to perform the designated clinical activities" (p. 90).

The issue of vicarious liability applies to the relationship that exists between the NP and the MCO as employer. Therefore, credentialing and privileging are necessary to ensure confidence in the ability to deliver quality patient care within the standards of practice (Younger et al., 1995). More information on vicarious liability was presented in Chapter 7.

DOCUMENTATION ISSUES IN MANAGED CARE

Personal Documentation Required
for Credentialing and Privileging

Documentation necessary for credentialing and privileging in an MCO requires the development of a continuously growing portfolio. Items that create the professional APN portfolio for privileging include experience with "disease prevention, health promotion, case management, utilization management, and risk management issues" (Rustia and Bartek, 1997, p. 99).

Documentation to Demonstrate Standards
of Performance

"It is no longer sufficient for the nurse to document that nursing care impacts positively on patient outcome; the nurse must also document that nursing care is the most cost-effective way of achieving the desired outcome" (Hicks, Stallmeyer, and Coleman, 1993, p. 42). The documenting of achievements at the end of planned nursing care is not merely an evaluation of the nursing care plan; it is the communication of benefits to having successful nursing interventions.

The American Nurses Association (1992) recognized that the actions of nurses often are multiple, episodic or continuous, fluid and varying, and less discrete than medical diagnostic categories. It is this diverse response to the care of patients that creates confusion in an evolving MCO that focuses on exact item-by-item responses to diseases or illnesses in its subscribers. Thus, the documentation issue is crucial for nurses to acknowledge, through the written medical record, the extent and breadth of services required to provide efficient resource allocation while coordinating care.

CONCLUSION

As MCOs proliferate throughout the United States, the emphasis on providing cost-effective care must be tempered with providing appropriate health care for individuals, not unidentified groups being managed according to a "cookbook" method. The future of MCOs is bright. Providing cost-efficient services by reducing overused and unnecessary diagnostic procedures and/or surgical procedures is a positive direction for health care delivery to take. Nursing can be an integral partner in providing primary care, home care, coordination services, and patient advocacy. Record keeping is an essential step in documenting the professional services and benefits derived from nursing services in the MCO environment of the 21st century.

A NATIONAL HEALTH INFORMATION SYSTEM FOR THE 21st CENTURY

DIALOGUE FOR A NATIONAL HEALTH INFORMATION SYSTEM

21

Sue E. Meiner
Elizabeth C. Mueth

Chapter Outline

The future of medical records that contain every element of a person's lifetime health care history is nearing reality. Computer-based records (CBRs) have made this a possibility within the current generation of Americans. This is an essential technological advance in the treatment of disease and the identification of statistical information from research for rapid dissemination to health care providers. Legal scrutiny of medical records will continue whenever negligence or malpractice in medicine is claimed. However, the restructuring of health care documentation with standardization of content, format, and language is now possible for the first time in the history of medical records. Computer technology and medical/nursing informatics have provided the essential tools to move forward.

Wenner (1998) found that 60% of all physician offices are equipped with computers. However, most are used for billing or scheduling purposes only. A national health information system (NHIS) requires that each primary health care provider have access to and routinely input medical data into a clinical information system. The NHIS can merge clinical and practice management systems into a national database.

Hospital and primary care offices are the most frequently observed areas for planning standardized databases. Outpatient records, including home health care (Chapter 16), have not been given much attention. Such medical records rarely are entered into a CBR system. According to Dick and Steen (1991), "Outpatient records are greater in number, are scattered among individual physician offices, and may exhibit even greater variance in quality than inpatient records. There are no established standards or review organizations for outpatient records as there are for inpatient records" (p. 19).

The proposed NHIS will be an integrated network linking government and private sector projects. New standards must be developed to permit interoperability. The existing standards such as ICD-0, ICD-9-CM, ICD-10, CPT (current procedural terminology), SNOWMED (systemized nomenclature of human and veterinary medicine), DRGs (diagnosis-related groups), *DSM-IV* (*Diagnostic and Statistical Manual,* fourth edition), READ codes, ICHPCC (international classification of health problems in primary care), CMIT (current medical information and technology), UNLS (Unified Nursing Language System), and UCDS (uniform clinical data set) nursing classifications must be integrated into a standard language. The Healthcare Informatics Standards Board of the American National Standards Institute coordinates standards among U.S. standards developers (Waegemann, 1998b).

A distinction must be made between CBRs (as discussed in Chapter 3) and computer-based accessible patient records (CBAPRs) in planning an NHIS. Whereas the CBR contains individual information of primary, secondary, and tertiary health care delivered by health care providers, the CBAPR relates to the information that the patient approves for access to health care providers. This affords each patient an opportunity to deny access to some or all of his or her individual health care records.

The issue of patient rights to privacy must be a consideration when the potential for complete and absolute access to individual health records is possible. This chapter presents information on the need for CBRs and CBAPRs as well as current problem areas that must be addressed prior to entering into an NHIS for all citizens of the United States.

NURSING PERSPECTIVE OF THE COMPUTER-BASED RECORD

Nursing documentation in the medical record is an example of an uncoordinated, fragmented system that often gives rise to discrepancies among entries concerning similar or identical elements of care within the same chart or record-keeping system that can lead to litigation. Shortliffe et al. (1992) concluded that "nurses spend an estimated 30[%] of their time documenting direct care given" (p. 276), and they discussed fragmentation of the patient's record by means of multiple forms maintained in multiple places within the health care environment. In acute care, the record might be at the bedside, in a central charting area within the nursing care unit, on departmental computer systems, or spread throughout all these places, with still additional information in a medical records central filing area.

Shortliffe et al. (1992) identified the repetitious nature of several areas of documentation that appear in different places in the chart, written by different health care workers, on different forms that pertain to the same data. They noted that text, image, and graphic records frequently were documented repeatedly. "This redundant data entry has the potential to result in erroneous entries, misdiagnosis, or mistreatment" (p. 277).

The CBR of the near future will need to address the issue of redundant information. Although the CBR can offer a comprehensive view of patient information, data should be entered only once for each component of patient care. The sophistication of computerized systems will afford the ability to retrieve data in multiple ways for different audiences. For example, when a nurse enters an abnormally elevated temperature once, an automatic, computer-driven trigger forwards this information to the physician, the pharmacy, the laboratory, and infection control alike.

A streamlined records system offers other benefits to the nurse as well, including decision-making support prompts, communication links with other departments within the facility, and statistics that can be used in risk management and quality improvement services. Patient teaching prompts and printed patient-specific teaching materials that address educational level and prior understanding of care are possible with computer systems with integrated programs. Discharge planning can link several services together for an efficient discharge procedure. Medications can be ready at the outpatient pharmacy, follow-up visits can be scheduled automatically, and instructions for home care can be printed on hard copy for both patient and family.

DISEASE OR TRAUMA TREATMENT AND COMPUTER-BASED RECORDS

Disease or trauma treatment using CBRs has the potential of providing up-to-the-minute research findings in all medical areas, especially in cancer and in neurological, heart, and respiratory diseases. A life-or-death condition has a very narrow window of time for medical/surgical decision making. Instantaneous information in critical time frames is a major benefit of easy access to CBRs. The health care provider must have accessible, intelligible clinical data pertaining to the current state of the patient and the patient's prior health management. Additional information from interactive decision support tools, based on data that have been analyzed for the treatment protocol, will enhance clinical decision making. The proposed plan of health management rests on rapid retrieval of such information from data storage systems.

EPIDEMIOLOGICAL IDENTIFICATION AND TREATMENT WITH COMPUTER-BASED RECORDS

Health departments throughout the United States have the task of identification, control, and prevention of health problems related to the environment and to infectious conditions. Thacker et al. (1996) reported the definition of public health surveillance as a continuous and organized collection of information on a defined health occurrence within the population under review. In addition, data analysis and interpretation must be disseminated to those professionals responsible for illness prevention and control.

Data obtained by public health agencies must be timely and representative of information that can be used in coordinating activities that will identify sentinel health events from environmental accidents or mismanagement or protect the public from epidemics of communicable disease. An example of environmental management is the discovery of dioxin in the soil in Times Beach, Missouri, in the 1980s. This mismanagement of chemical disposal caused an entire town to be disbanded and all its buildings to be destroyed. Communicable disease identification and prevention of the spread of disease are other emergent events.

Obtaining information from data sources can be difficult when records are maintained in local offices in unitary form. A CBR system that can automatically send coded communicable disease information to a central collection source, such as the Centers for Disease Control and Prevention in Atlanta, Georgia, is beneficial to the entire citizenry.

PERSONAL PRIVACY AND COMPUTER RECORDS

A major concern of the American people with regard to a computer-based documentation system is personal privacy. At a time when nearly everything that is purchased is recorded on a computer and when those data seem available to nearly anyone willing to buy the privilege, personal privacy in the United States is in jeopardy.

The Privacy Act of 1974 provides assurance to the public that patient records under the jurisdiction of the federal government will not be disclosed to third parties, except under defined circumstances, without the consent of the patient.

Most states have enacted laws that safeguard personal privacy and health records but do not include privacy protection to third-party payers, insurance companies, or (in some cases) employers (Waller, 1991).

When health care records are requested for nonmedical purposes, most laws are not thorough enough to fully protect privacy rights. Waller (1991) noted, "Most states expressly allow a patient or a patient's authorized representative to inspect and copy the patient's hospital records. Rights of access to health records maintained by physicians and other health care providers may not always be clear" (p. 165).

Security can be maintained in the NHIS by keeping CBRs for each locality stored regionally and linked via a national network rather than creating a single national database. Local CBR systems would have all of the original security systems and fire walls in place and would be accessible only by permission from each individual patient, or legal representative, through the use of authorization codes.

Disclosure of Health Data and
the Computer-Based Accessible Patient Record

When medical information is needed for diagnostic and treatment reasons, the information should be accessible by those medical persons needing to know so as to make a correct diagnosis. If, however, certain components of an individual's past medical record are not needed for the current treatment, then should they be made available anyway? This question must be answered prior to all health care records being submitted to regional or even national information systems' data banks.

When specific health events in a person's past give cause for personal, family, cultural, or environmental concerns or embarrassment, thought must be given to the *need to know* of anyone except the initial health care provider. The choice to permit access to prior health care records needs to be made with informed consent, not with a blanket permission to access all records. The patient should be given the reason for the need to obtain all old health records prior to any request that they be made available.

Informed consent for personalized accessibility to health care records can be given with fire walls that provide multiple levels of consent. Some levels may permit specific health care providers to access part or all of the CBAPR, whereas access can be narrow in scope with significant limitations. Narrow access could reduce potential legal liability where the lack of information contributed to misdiagnosis or mistreatment episodes.

According to the provisions of the Kennedy-Kassebaum bill, each patient in the NHIS must have a unique identifier (Appavu, 1998). Many technologies may be used to fulfill this mandate. Identity cards may be plastic, paper, or optical. They may have unique identifying numbers or codes, bar codes, graphic codes, magnetic stripes, or chips (smart cards). Patient identity cards can assist with many functions such as patient identification, coverage eligibility, insurance, professional identification, health passport, and/or follow-up cards. Card installations have been successfully installed in Germany, France, Italy, Spain, and the United Kingdom (Waegemann, 1998a).

COMPROMISING PRIVACY VERSUS COMPROMISING HEALTH CARE

The right to personal privacy is an American expectation. That expectation extends to confidentiality of medical records. Confidentiality addresses not only prevention of unauthorized viewing of the health records but also restriction of disclosure of past treatment for conditions unrelated to the reason for seeking current health care attention. Donaldson and Lohr (1994) noted, "Other parties external to the healing relationship seek person-identified information and assert socially beneficial reasons for access" (p. 141). They identified groups that have made the medical record of individuals part of their business. These groups include government entitlement programs; attorneys who are investigating charges against agencies or health care providers; and agencies that protect children, spouses, and the elderly from abuse. The personal privacy issue regarding access to individuals' medical records, especially when computer access is available, should be approached as an informed consent matter.

Several lifestyle issues that influence health care are tobacco use, alcohol use, mental illnesses, sexually transmitted diseases, HIV, and family history of genetic disease. If personal privacy issues prevent such information from reaching the attention of health care providers, then factors influencing the overall health and well-being of individuals and even the public generally could be at stake. Donaldson and Lohr (1994) stated, "The more detailed the information about an individual or [a] class of individuals, the more appropriate, one hopes, is the treatment they will be given. Further[more], documentation of care and risk factors are essential to promoting continuity of care over time and among providers" (pp. 140-141). When health data are limited or incomplete, the risks of misdiagnosis or errors in clinical decision making are magnified.

Seeking Consent to Access Health-Related Data

According to Bulger (1994), "Protection of the individual record from person-identifiable exposure must involve all possible behavioral, systematic, and technical security measures" (p. vi). Without consent, invasions of privacy can occur when an intentional breach results from unauthorized access to personal information. In the medical records context, privacy turns on the interest of an individual in controlling the access and use of personal information.

Powers (1991) discussed informational privacy as maintaining personal data without permitting access to those data by others through reading, listening, or using any of the human senses. Westin (1967) described privacy and freedom as "the claim of individuals, groups, or institutions to determine for themselves when, how, and to what extent information about them is communicated to others" (p. 7). Westin's definition provided the foundation for the Privacy Act.

CONCLUSION

Standardized computer language for data entry will bring about uniform data collection and will promote data integrity. Data collected in the NHIS repositories may then be analyzed for epidemiological studies.

Care must be taken to comply with Health Information Portability and Accountability Act legislation, Health Care Financing Administration regulations, and state legislation. Such legislation identifies specific security requirements to protect health information (Lovorn, 1998). Policies and procedures must be in place to govern access control and the use of authorization codes and electronic signatures including provisions for secondary charting codes.

Existing data systems that can form the basis for an NHIS need to be identified. New modes of information systems that can be added to existing systems are needed to complete a workable NHIS. This process of information systems development must be addressed in an aggressive manner through the formation of local and regional focus groups that can identify routine and special information needs for patient records. These focus group teams need to have a multidisciplinary membership with representation from each of the areas that contributes to the medical record. Meetings should be scheduled to review existing information system programs with the most comprehensive formats. Recommendation for additions, deletions, and/or changes to the best information system programs should follow, with the resulting documentation system tested in a variety of pilot projects.

Patient rights issues will continue to be a concern for U.S. citizens as computer technology in health care continues to progress. The interest in personal autonomy through information privacy is vital to a sense of well-being in most Americans. Loss of privacy will provide an opportunity for various groups to apply unrestrained control over an individual's economic, personal, and psychosocial well-being. Access to personal medical records must be viewed as an issue of informed consent. To ensure patient privacy, providers will have access only to information needed for the immediate health care treatment. Patients will give permission for access to selected CBR systems or records (CBAPRs).

Privacy advocates will continue to watch for breaching of databases that go beyond the integrated CBR or CBAPR. These advocates will need to watch for problems inherent in merging of financial, credit, and lifestyle information systems. The fear of privacy loss due to a national identification database of every citizen should serve as reason to participate in a national multidisciplinary task force to oversee issues of privacy in medical CBRs as the health care industry and the nation work toward an NHIS to maintain the highest quality health care in the world.

SAMPLES

COLLABORATIVE PRACTICE AGREEMENT
(for use with advanced practice nurses)

This Collaborative Practice Agreement entered into this ____ day of
_____, 199__, by and between _____, a physician duly
licensed to practice medicine in the State of Missouri (hereinafter "Physician")
and an advanced practice nurse as defined in Section 335.016(2) R.S.Mo. (1993)
(hereinafter "APN").

Physician, having reviewed APN's skill training and competence, hereby
delegates to APN the authority to administer, dispense, and prescribe drugs and
provide treatment within the APN's scope of practice and consistent with APN's
skill, training, and competence. The forgoing delegation to APN to prescribe
drugs shall exclude the prescribing of controlled substances but shall include the
administration and dispensing of controlled drugs. There is incorporated herein
and made a part hereof, protocols which have been jointly agreed upon by
Physician and APN and/or standing orders issued by Physician. The protocols
and/or standing orders may be added to or modified from time to time. Such
protocols and/or standing orders must be written, signed, and dated by Physician
prior to their implementation.

By this delegation, and, pursuant to Section 338.198 R.S.Mo. (1993), APN
is permitted to authorize pharmacists to fill prescriptions, including telephone
prescriptions as defined in Section 338.095.2 R.S.Mo. (1993). Such prescriptions
may be forwarded or transmitted to the pharmacist by the APN, a registered
professional nurse, a registered physician's assistant, or other authorized agent.

This Collaborative Practice Agreement is good only for the following
locations and/or facilities: _____. This Collaborative Practice Agreement and the delegation of authority herein may be revoked at any time upon
written notice from Physician to APN. The APN may terminate this Agreement
at any time upon written notice to Physician.

PHYSICIAN   APN

_____   _____

_____   _____

(DATE)   (DATE)

SOURCE: Developed by the Missouri Society of Hospital Attorneys for the Missouri Hospital Association, 1993.
Used with permission. Sample only—This form should be used only upon consultation with legal counsel.

EMPLOYMENT AGREEMENT

This employment agreement is entered into this ____ day of _____, 199__, by and between _____ (partnership, corporation, or individual) and _____, an advanced practice nurse (hereinafter "APN"), where APN is an employee of _____. This agreement shall be effective as of _____, 199__.

The estimated start date of employment is _____, 199__.

The following conditions of employment apply:

1. The full-time (36-40 hours per week) rate of pay will be _____ (stated as dollar amount) per _____ (specify hour, week, pay period, year) plus 10 percent of net practice revenues.
2. Practice overhead costs to be paid by _____.
3. State RN/APN license renewal fees to be paid by _____. DEA [Drug Enforcement Agency] registration and renewal fees to be paid by _____.
4. Professional association fees up to, but not to exceed, $500 per year to be paid by _____.
5. Professional journal and publication subscription fees up to, but not to exceed, $500 per year to be paid by _____.
6. CME [continuing medical education] costs up to, but not to exceed, $1,500 per year to be paid by _____.
7. Medical, hospitalization, dental, and vision insurance premiums to be paid by _____. Dependent and family medical, hospitalization, dental, and vision insurance premiums to be paid by _____.
8. Life insurance and short- and long-term disability premiums to be paid by _____.
9. Malpractice insurance to be paid by _____.
10. Profit-sharing and 401k benefits will be paid at _____ percent by _____.
11. Mileage calculated at the current government rate to be paid monthly by _____, and associated travel expenses to be paid by _____.
12. APN to be included in any marketing strategies (including advertisements, brochures, business cards, etc.) to be used to promote practice. In addition, APN to be allocated $1,000 annually for advertising expenses.
13. APN's performance to be reviewed every three (3) months and evaluated in writing every six (6) months. Performance review and evaluation shall be based upon, but not limited to, quality of care, patient satisfaction, chart review, peer review, and productivity. Merit raises of _____ percent of annual salary to be given upon positive performance appraisal every _____ months.
14. Cost-of-living increases based on annual inflation rate to be given yearly upon anniversary date of hire.

15. Yearly bonuses of up to 15 percent of base salary to be paid according to the following formula: 5 percent if practice is profitable; 5 percent based on meeting a threshold* of patient visits; and 5 percent based on patient satisfaction, staff satisfaction, and citizenship. (*Threshold is defined as _____ patient visits per _____ [amount of time].)

16. Paid vacation time of _____ days per year, to be taken at APN's discretion. Unused vacation time to be carried over to subsequent year(s) or paid out annually at APN's option.

17. Paid sick time or paid personal-time-off of _____ days per year. Unused sick or personal-time-off days to be carried over to subsequent year(s) or paid out annually at APN's option.

18. Paid CME time of _____ days per year, to be taken at APN's discretion.

19. Paid holidays will include New Year's Day, Memorial Day, Fourth of July, Labor Day, Thanksgiving, Christmas, and APN's birthday.

20. Termination of employment by either party shall require a 30-day written notice.

The following parties agree to the stipulations of this employment agreement.

_____   _____
APN   Date   Name/Title   Date

SOURCE: Diane E. Dito and Louise L. Kidd. Used with permission.

NURSE PRACTITIONER/PHYSICIAN
COLLABORATIVE PRACTICE AGREEMENT

This collaborative practice agreement (hereinafter referred to as "Agreement") is entered into this _____ day of _____, 19__, by and between _____, a physician duly licensed to practice medicine in the State of _____ (hereinafter referred to as "Physician"), and _____, a registered professional nurse in the State of _____, who is also recognized by the _____ State Board of Nursing as an Advanced Practice Nurse (hereinafter referred to as "APN"), and shall be effective commencing on _____, 19__.

The purpose of this Agreement is to reflect the understanding that has been developed and the relationship that exists between APN and Physician. This Agreement delegates authority to APN to perform specific medical acts as outlined herein. Physician hereby delegates to APN the authority to administer, dispense, and prescribe medications and provide treatment within APN's scope of practice and consistent with APN's skill, training, and competence. The forgoing delegation to APN to prescribe medications shall exclude the prescribing of controlled substances but shall include the administration and dispensing of controlled medications. By this delegation, and pursuant to Section 338.098 R.S.Mo. (1993), APN is permitted to authorize a pharmacist to fill prescriptions on behalf of Physician, including telephone prescriptions, as defined in Section 338.095.2 R.S.Mo. (1993). This Agreement is not intended to be restrictive and may be amended by agreement of Physician and APN to delegate authority to perform additional medical acts according to any additional education, training, and/or certification APN may obtain. This Agreement does not apply to APN's independent practice of nursing but rather to those delegated medical acts listed herein and those nursing acts which require physician orders.

I. General Information

    A. APN

        Name: _____

        State License Number: _____

        Area of Certification: _____

        Certification Number: _____

        Certifying Organization: _____

        Expiration Date: _____

    B. Physician and Designated Covering Physician(s)

        Name: _____

        State Registration Number: _____

        Board Certification Area: _____

Name: _____

State Registration Number: _____

Board Certification Area: _____

C. Description of Setting of APN

    1. Type of Setting(s)

    The APN practices in the _____

    at _____ .

    The APN also practices at _____ ,

    a _____ .

    2. Type and Volume of Patients

    (LIST: anticipated volume of patients seen in setting annually, age groups, number of physicals, procedures, etc., expected to be performed per day, type of clients seen, and any other pertinent information.)

II. Nurse Practitioner Functions

In this practice, APN may perform the following functions (if YES, please describe terms and conditions of each item).

A. Obtain history and perform comprehensive physical assessment of patients.

    YES ____   NO ____

B. Establish medical diagnoses for common short-term or chronic, stable health problems.

    YES ____   NO ____

    Common short-term or chronic, stable health problems may be diagnosed and treated by the APN independently with consultation of Physician as necessary.

C. Order, perform, and/or interpret laboratory tests.

    YES ____   NO ____

    APN may, independently or with Physician collaboration, order, perform, and interpret laboratory tests, consistent with APN's training and scope of practice.

D. Order, perform, and/or interpret diagnostic tests (X-ray, CT [computerized tomography], ultrasound, and MRI [magnetic resonance imaging]).

    YES ____   NO ____

APN may, independently or with Physician collaboration, order, perform, and interpret diagnostic tests, consistent with APN's training and scope of practice.

E. Perform specific invasive procedures.

YES ____   NO ____

Invasive procedures performed by APN independently or with Physician consult are listed below. APN has successfully completed the didactic, instructional, and/or performance criteria and has demonstrated competency for each invasive procedure listed.

1. (LIST), etc.

F. Tests/procedures performed only by the physician are as listed below.

1. (LIST), etc.

G. Prescribe medications.

YES ____   NO ____

APN may prescribe noncontrolled substances independently or in collaboration with Physician. The APN shall not under any circumstances prescribe controlled medications but may administer and dispense such medications per physician order. Noncontrolled medications the APN may prescribe include but are not limited to:

1. (LIST), etc.

H. Order and/or perform therapeutic or corrective treatments.

YES ____   NO ____

Therapeutic or corrective measures the APN may order and/or perform include but are not limited to:

1. (LIST), etc.

I. Refer patients to appropriate licensed physicians and other health care providers.

YES ____   NO ____

Referrals are made to physicians and other health care providers as appropriate and deemed necessary. Referrals may be made independently or in collaboration with Physician or his/her designate. These may include social service, dentistry, mental health, hearing and speech agencies, gynecology, obstetrics, cardiology, neurology, endocrinology, psychiatry, orthopedics, dermatology, hematology, surgical, allergy, genetics, etc.

III. Miscellaneous Provisions

    A. This Agreement shall be effective from _____ (MM/DD/YY) until _____ (MM/DD/YY). If both parties desire to renew this Agreement at the end of the stated term, the Agreement shall be renegotiated on or before _____ (MM/DD/YY). This Agreement and the delegation of authority herein may be terminated by either party by notifying the other party at least 30 days prior to the proposed termination date.

    B. Physician and APN agree that any and all rights, obligations, or authority provided by this written contract are personal to them and that neither party may assign or transfer to any other person or persons such rights, obligations, or authority without prior written consent of the other party.

    C. This Agreement may be modified at any time by written agreement signed by both parties or superseded by execution of a new agreement signed by both parties.

    D. Physician and APN shall maintain for a minimum of eight (8) years upon termination of this Agreement their own personal copies of this Agreement, all amendments, any applicable protocols and standing orders, and any notice of termination of this Agreement.

    E. APN's performance will be reviewed by Physician or his/her designee every three (3) months and evaluated in writing every six (6) months. Performance review and evaluation shall be based upon, but not limited to, quality of care, patient satisfaction, chart review, peer review, and productivity.

Signature and date of signature shall be affixed by all parties entering into this Agreement.

_____

APN   Date   Physician   Date

SOURCE: Diane E. Dito and Louise L. Kidd. Used with permission.

AMERICAN ASSOCIATION OF LEGAL NURSE CONSULTING CHAPTERS (AS OF 1998)

Headquarters

> 4700 West Lake Avenue
> Glenview, IL 60025-1485
> Phone: (847) 375-4713
> Fax: (847) 375-4777

Arizona

> Phoenix Chapter
> P.O. Box 13441
> Phoenix, AZ 85002

California

> Bay Area of Northern California
> P.O. Box 3300
> San Leandro, CA 94578-0300

> Los Angeles Chapter
> P.O. Box 9222
> Whittier, CA 90608-9222

> Orange County Chapter of Southern California
> 5405 Alton Parkway, Suite 5A450
> Irvine, CA 92604

> Greater Sacramento Area Chapter
> P.O. Box 660011
> Sacramento, CA 95866-0011

> San Diego Chapter
> P.O. Box 2822
> San Diego, CA 92112-2822

Delaware

Diamond State Chapter
P.O. Box 4265
Greenville, DE 19807

Florida

Greater Fort Lauderdale Chapter
P.O. Box 698
Fort Lauderdale, FL 33302

Miami Chapter
P.O. Box 110134
Miami, FL 33111-0134

Greater Orlando Chapter
P.O. Box 3201
Orlando, FL 32802-3201

Georgia

Atlanta Chapter
P.O. Box 55438
Atlanta, GA 30308

Illinois

Greater Chicago Chapter
P.O. Box A-3913
Chicago, IL 60690

Indiana

Greater Indianapolis Chapter
P.O. Box 1702
Indianapolis, IN 46206-1702

Kentucky

Lexington/Kentucky Chapter
P.O. Box 22535
Lexington, KY 40522-2535

Louisiana

Baton Rouge Chapter
3216 West Esplanade, A4-288
Metarie, LA 70005

Maryland

Greater Baltimore Area Chapter
P.O. Box 342112
Bethesda, MD 20827-2112

Michigan

Greater Detroit Chapter
P.O. Box 1
Chelsea, MI 48118

Minnesota

Minneapolis Chapter
P.O. Box 2843
Minneapolis, MN 55402

Missouri

St. Louis Chapter
P.O. Box 50166
Clayton, MO 63105

New York

Rochester/New York Chapter
P.O. Box 92204
Rochester, NY 14692

Ohio

Cleveland/NEO Chapter
P.O. Box 455
Chesterland, OH 44072

Youngstown/Ohio Chapter
7100 Lockwood Blvd., Suite 183
Youngstown, OH 44512

Oregon

> Greater Portland/Valley Chapter
> 1500 Gossamere Lane
> Stayton, OR 97383

Pennsylvania

> Philadelphia Chapter
> 175 Strafford Avenue, Suite 1
> Wayne, PA 19087
>
> Pittsburgh Chapter
> P.O. Box 97104
> Pittsburgh, PA 15229-0104

Rhode Island

> Greater Providence Chapter
> 8 Country Drive
> Hingham, MA 02043

South Carolina

> Columbia Chapter
> P.O. Box 1866
> Columbia, SC 29202-1866

Texas

> Austin Chapter
> P.O. Box 5294
> Austin, TX 78763
>
> Dallas Chapter
> P.O. Box 50394
> Dallas, TX 75250
>
> Fort Worth Chapter
> P.O. Box 866
> Fort Worth, TX 76101
>
> Greater Houston Chapter
> 7500 San Felipe, Suite 600
> Houston, TX 77063

REFERENCES

Agency for Health Care Policy and Research: *Clinical practice guidelines: Pressure ulcer treatment.* Pub. No. 15. Rockville, MD: U.S. Department of Health and Human Services, 1994.

Agency for Health Care Policy and Research: *Managing acute and chronic urinary incontinence.* Publication No. 96-0686. Rockville, MD: U.S. Department of Health and Human Services, 1996.

Aguilera DC: *Crisis intervention: Theory and methodology.* 8th ed. St. Louis, MO: C. V. Mosby, 1997.

Ahmann E: Family centered care: The time has come. *Pediatric Nursing* 20 (1): 52-53, 1994.

Alspach JG: Core curriculum for critical care nursing. In *Legal and ethical aspects of critical care nursing,* 4th ed., GS Woody, ed. Philadelphia: W. B. Saunders, 1991, pp. 905-926.

American Academy of Nurse Practitioners: *Nurse practitioner tips for contracting.* Washington, DC: Author, n.d.

American Academy of Nurse Practitioners: *The nurse practitioner in managed care organizations.* Austin, TX: Author, 1997.

American Nurses Association: *Code for nurses with interpretive statements.* Kansas City, MO: Author, 1985.

American Nurses Association: *Nursing facts.* Washington, DC: Author, 1992.

American Nurses Association: *A statement on psychiatric-mental health clinical nursing practice and standards of psychiatric/mental health clinical nursing practice.* Washington, DC: Author, 1994.

American Nurses Association: *Nursing's social policy statement.* Washington, DC: Author, 1995.

American Nurses Credentialing Center: *Recertification requirements: General information.* Washington, DC: American Nurses Association, 1997.

American Psychiatric Association: *Report of the Task Force on Psychiatric Uses of Seclusion and Restraint.* Washington, DC: Author, 1985.

Appavu SI: Healthcare identifiers [abstract]. In *Toward an electronic patient record '98.* Newton, MA: Medical Records Institute, 1998.

Appleby C: Boxed in? *Hospital Health Network* 69 (18): 28-30, 32, 34, 1995a.

Appleby C: HMOs on the move: Is your town big enough for the both of you? *Hospital Health Network* 69 (22): 28-32, 1995b.

Association of Operating Room Nurses: *AORN standards and recommended practices for perioperative nursing 1998.* Denver, CO: Author, 1998.

Association of Women's Health, Obstetric, and Neonatal Nurses: *Standards for the nursing care of women and newborns.* 4th ed. Washington, DC: Author, 1994.

Atkinson L and Fortunato N: Legal and ethical issues. In *Berry & Kohn's operating room technique,* L Atkinson and N Fortunado, eds. St. Louis, MO: C. V. Mosby, 1996, pp. 53-55.

Becker PA: Legal issues for nurses: Overview of professional liability insurance. *Texas Nursing* 67 (6): 13, 1993.

Beckmann J: *Nursing negligence: Analyzing malpractice in the hospital setting.* Thousand Oaks, CA: Sage, 1996.

Bernzweig E: *The nurse's liability for malpractice: A programmed course.* 6th ed. St. Louis, MO: C. V. Mosby, 1996.

Besharov DJ: Policy guidelines for decision making in child abuse and neglect. *Child Today* 16 (6): 7-10, 33, 1987.

Black HC: *Black's law dictionary.* St. Paul, MN: West, 1991.

Bosk CL: *Forgive and remember: Managing medical failure.* Chicago: University of Chicago Press, 1981.

Bostrom J and Suter WN: Charge nurse decision making about patient assignment. *Nursing Administration Quarterly* 16 (4): 32-38, 1992.

Branson FL: *Handling the ob-gyn case.* San Antonio: Texas Tech University Law School Foundation, 1996.

Brent NJ: *Nurses and the law.* Philadelphia: W. B. Saunders, 1997.

Bryant H and Fernald L: Nursing knowledge and use of restraint alternatives: Acute and chronic care. *Geriatric Nursing* 18 (2): 57, 1997.

Buckley-Womack C and Gidney B: A new dimension in documentation: The PIE method. *Journal of Neuroscience Nursing* 19 (3): 256-260, 1987.

Bulger RJ: Preface. In *Health data in the information age: Use, disclosure, and privacy,* M Donaldson and K Lohr, eds. Washington, DC: National Academy Press, 1994.

Burke LJ and Murphy J: *Charting by exception: A cost-effective quality approach.* New York: John Wiley, 1995.

Byars WB: Legal challenges created by computerized medical records. *Topics in Health Information Management* 16 (4): 61-65, 1996.

Chase SK: Charting critical thinking: Nursing judgments and patient outcomes. *Dimensions of Critical Care Nursing* 16 (2): 102-111, 1997.

Darovic GO: *Introduction to the care of critically ill and injured patients.* 2nd ed. Philadelphia: W. B. Saunders, 1995.

Daudell-Strejc D and Murphy C: Emerging clinical issues in home health psychiatric nursing. *Home Healthcare Nurse* 13: 17, 1995.

Davino M: You don't have to care for every patient. *RN* 59 (9): 63-67, 1996.

Diamond JL, Lawrence CL, and Madden MS: *Understanding torts.* New York: Matthew Bender, 1996.

Dick R and Steen E: *The computer-based patient record: An essential technology for health care.* Washington, DC: National Academy Press, 1991.

Donaldson M and Lohr K: *Health data in the information age: Use, disclosure, and privacy.* Washington, DC: National Academy Press, 1994.

Dunkel RM: Parish nurses help patients: Body and soul. *RN* 59 (5): 55-56, 1996.

Dykes PC and Wheeler K: *Planning, implementing, and evaluating critical pathways: A guide for health care survival into the 21st century.* New York: Springer, 1997.

Ebersole P and Hess P: *Toward healthy aging: Human needs and nursing response.* 5th ed. St. Louis, MO: C. V. Mosby, 1998.

Edmunds M: Time of risk, time of opportunity. *The Nurse Practitioner* 19 (8): 7-8, 11, 1994.

Eggland ET: Making the transition to home health care charting. *Nursing 96* 26 (3): 16, 1996.

Eggland ET: Charting tips. *Nursing 97,* 27 (1): 17, 1997.

Emergency Nurses Association: *ENA: Standards of practice.* 2nd ed. St. Louis, MO: C. V. Mosby, 1991a.

Emergency Nurses Association: Telephone advice. *Journal of Emergency Nursing* 17: 52, 1991b.

Facione NC and Facione PA: Assessment design issues for evaluating critical thinking in nursing. *Holistic Nursing Practice* 10 (3): 41-53, 1996.

Fairchild S: Legal aspects of perioperative nursing practice. In *Perioperative nursing principles and practice,* S Fairchild, ed. Boston: Jones & Bartlett, 1993, pp. 367-370.

Fitzmaurice JM, Murphy G, Wear P, Korpman R, Weber G, and Whiteman J: Patient identifiers: Stumbling blocks or cornerstones for CPRs? *Healthcare Informatics* 10 (5): 38-40, 1993.

Fogg DM: Clinical issues: Patient positioning. *AORN Journal* 58 (6): 1192-1193, 1993.

Foltz D: Long-term care national database. *Medical Record Newsletter* (November), 1994.

Foreman JT: Continuous quality improvement in home care. *Caring* 12 (10): 32-37, 1993.

Friedman E: Dysfunctional labor. In *Obstetrics,* 13th ed., JP Greenhill, ed. Philadelphia: W. B. Saunders, 1965.

Garbarino J, Guttmann E, and Seeley J: *The psychologically battered child.* San Francisco: Jossey-Bass, 1986.

Gardner RA: Belated realization of child sex abuse by an adult. *Issues in Child Abuse Accusations* 4 (4): 177-195, 1992.

Gilham CS: Legal implications of computerized medical records. *Health Progress* 77 (3), 18-19, 1996.

Giuliano K and Poirier C: Nursing case management: Critical pathways to desirable patient outcomes. *Nursing Management* 22 (3): 52, 1991.

Goldrick B and Larson E: Wound management in home care: An assessment. *Journal of Community Health Nursing* 10 (1), 23-29, 1993.

Grant AE: Documenting by computer. *Nursing 93,* 23 (9): 53, 1993.

Gray-Miceli D: Evaluation and treatment of falls. *Advances for Nurse Practitioners* 3 (11): 29, 1995.

Guard R and Langman MM: Legislative priorities for medical libraries: Computerized patient records. *MLA News* 301: 22, 1997.

Guido GW: *Legal issues in nursing.* 2nd ed. Stamford, CT: Appleton & Lange, 1997.

Hamric A, Spross J, and Hanson C (Eds.): *Advanced nursing practice: Integrative approach.* Philadelphia: W. B. Saunders, 1996.

Hansen R and Washburn M: Tips for delegating to the right person. *American Journal of Nursing* 26 (6): 64-65, 1992.

Health Care Financing Administration: *Medicare home health agency manual publication 11.* Washington, DC: Author, 1989.

Health Care Financing Administration: *Survey, certification, and enforcement procedures.* Baltimore, MD: Author, 1994.

Health Care Financing Administration: *Resident assessment instrument training manual and resource guide.* Baltimore, MD: Author, 1995.

Hendrich A: *Falls, immobility, and restraints: Staff education handbook.* St. Louis, MO: C. V. Mosby, 1996.

Hershey N: Student, instructor, and liability. *American Journal of Nursing* 65 (3): 122-123, 1965.

Hicks LL, Stallmeyer JM, and Coleman JR: *Role of the nurse in managed care.* Washington, DC: American Nurses Association, 1993.

Holmberg S: A walking program for wanderers: Volunteer training and development of an evening walker's group. *Geriatric Nursing* 18 (3): 120, 1997.

Huber D: *Leadership and nursing care management.* Philadelphia: W. B. Saunders, 1996.

Humphrey C and Milone-Nuzzo P: *Orientation to home care nursing.* Gaithersburg, MD: Aspen, 1996.

Iyer P: Thirteen charting rules to keep you legally safe. *Nursing 91,* 21 (6): 40-45, 1991.

Iyer P: Computer charting: Minimizing legal risks. *Nursing 93* 23 (5): 86, 1993.

Iyer P and Camp N: *Nursing documentation: A nursing process approach.* 2nd ed. St. Louis, MO: C. V. Mosby, 1995.

Johnson BA and Niederman GA: *Managed care legal issues: A practical guide for health care decision-makers.* Englewood, CO: Medical Group Management Association, 1996.

Joint Commission on Accreditation of Healthcare Organizations: *Standards for the accreditation of home care.* Chicago: Author, 1993.

Joint Commission on Accreditation of Healthcare Organizations: *Accreditation manual for hospitals.* Oakbrook Terrace, IL: Author, 1995.

Joint Commission on Accreditation of Healthcare Organizations: *1997 hospital accreditation standards.* Oakbrook Terrace, IL: Author, 1996.

Kadzielski MA and Reynolds MB: Legal review: Auto-authentication of medical records raised verification concerns. *Topics in Health Information Management* 14 (1): 77-82, 1993.

Kalisch PA and Kalisch BJ: The press image of community health nurses, *Public Health Nursing,* March 1, 1984, pp. 3-15.

Kane RL, Ouslander JG, and Abrass IB: Instability and falls. In *Essentials of clinical geriatrics,* RL Kane, JG Ouslander, and IB Abrass, eds. New York: McGraw-Hill, 1994, pp. 197-219.

Keeton PW: *Prosser and Keeton on the law of torts.* 5th ed. St. Paul, MN: West, 1984.

Kerr SD: A comparison of four nursing documentation systems. *Journal of Nursing Staff Development* 8 (1): 27-31, 1992.

Ketter J: The ethical and legal implications of restructuring. *The American Nurse* 26 (7): 23, 1994.

Kibbe D and Bard MR: How safe are computerized patient records? *Family Practice Management,* May, 1997. (Available on Internet: http://www.aafp.org/fpm/970500fm/lead/html)

Kidd PS and Wagner KD: *High acuity nursing.* 2nd ed. Stamford, CT: Appleton & Lange, 1996.

King MB and Tinetti ME: Falls in community-dwelling older persons. *Journal of the American Geriatrics Society* 43: 1146-1154, 1995.

Kneedler JA and Dodge GH: *Perioperative patient care: The nursing perspective.* 2nd ed. Sudbury, MA: Jones & Bartlett, 1991.

Kraus GP: *Healthcare risk management.* Owings Mills, MD: Rynd Communications, National Health Publishing, 1986.

Kravitz RL, Rolph JE, and McGuigan K: Malpractice claims data as a quality improvement tool. I. Epidemiology of error in four specialties. *Journal of the American Medical Association* 266: 2087, 1991.

Kreitzer W: Legal aspects of child abuse: Guidelines for the nurse. *Nursing Clinics of North America* 16 (1): 149, 1981.

Krugman R: Advances and retreats in the protection of children. *New England Journal of Medicine* 320 (8): 531-532, 1989a.

Krugman R: New light on a dark area: An update on child abuse and neglect. *Current Opinions in Pediatrics* 1 (1): 168-171, 1989b.

La Puma J and Schiedermayer D: *Pocket guide to managed care: Business, practice, law, ethics.* New York: McGraw-Hill, 1996.

Lanros NE and Barber JM: *Emergency nursing.* 4th ed. Stamford, CT: Appleton & Lange, 1997.

Latz PA: Computerized nursing documentation systems. *AORN Journal* 56 (2): 300-311, 1992.

Lee PR and Estes CL: *The nation's health.* 5th ed. Sudbury, MA: Jones & Bartlett, 1997.

Lepler M: Floating. *Revolution* 3 (1), 10-12, 14, 16, 1993.

Lovejoy D: *Making the transition to home health nursing: A practical guide.* New York: Springer, 1997.

Lovorn J: Healthcare identifiers [abstract]. In *Toward an electronic patient record '98.* Newton, MA: Medical Records Institute, 1998.

Lueckenotte AG: *Gerontologic nursing.* St. Louis, MO: C. V. Mosby, 1996.

Luggen AS, Travis SS, and Meiner SE (Eds.): *NGNA core curriculum for gerontological advanced practice nurses.* Thousand Oaks, CA: Sage, 1998.

Lyons TK and Payne BD: The relationship of physicians' medical recording performance to their medical care performance. *Medical Care* 12 (8): 714-720, 1974.

Marrelli TM: *Handbook of home health standards and documentation guidelines for reimbursement.* 2nd ed. St. Louis, MO: C. V. Mosby, 1994.

Mattson S and Smith JE: *NAACOG core curriculum for maternal-newborn nursing.* Philadelphia: W. B. Saunders, 1993.

McCloskey JC and Grace HK: *Current issues in nursing.* St. Louis, MO: C. V. Mosby, 1990.

Meeker MH and Rothrock JC: *Alexander's care of the patient in surgery.* 10th ed. St. Louis, MO: C. V. Mosby, 1997.

Meisel A and Kuczewski M: Legal and ethical myths about informed consent. *Archives of Internal Medicine* 156: 2521-2526, 1996.

Mezey M and McGivern D: *Nurses, nurse practitioners: Evolution to advanced practice.* New York: Springer, 1993.

Milholland DK and Heiler BR: The computer-based patient record. In *Information management in nursing and health care,* MEC Mills, CA Romano, and BR Heller, eds. Springhouse, PA: Springhouse Corporation, 1996.

Miller BF and Keane CB: *Miller-Keane encyclopedia and dictionary of medicine, nursing, and allied health.* 6th ed. Philadelphia: W. B. Saunders, 1997.

Miller T: Political involvement and community health advocacy. In *Community health nursing: Concepts and practice,* BS Spradley, ed. Boston: Little, Brown, 1990.

Missouri Nurses Association: Assignment despite objection. *Missouri Nurse* 65 (4): 9, 1996.

Missouri Nurses Association: *Collaborative practice agreement* [brochure]. Jefferson City: Author, 1997.

Murphy EK: Legal ramifications of RN staffing policies. *AORN Journal* 59 (5): 1064, 1067-68, 1070, 1994.

Nurses Association of the American Academy of Obstetricians and Gynecologists: *The nurse's role in induction/augmentation of labor.* Washington, DC: Author, 1988.

National Association for Home Care: *Basic statistics about home care.* Washington, DC: Author, 1996.

National Council of State Boards of Nursing: *Position paper on the regulation of advanced nursing practice.* Chicago: Author, 1993.

National Council of State Boards of Nursing: *Delegation: Concepts and decision-making process.* Chicago: Author, 1995.

National Institute on Aging: *Special report on aging.* Bethesda, MD: U.S. Department of Health and Human Services, Public Health Service, 1990.

Nicholls DJ, Duplaga EA, and Meyer LM: Nurses' attitudes about floating. *Nursing Management* 27 (1): 56-58, 1996.

North American Nursing Diagnosis Association: *Taxonomy I revised with official nursing diagnoses.* St. Louis, MO: Author, 1990.

Northrup CE and Kelly ME: *Legal issues in nursing.* St. Louis, MO: C. V. Mosby, 1987.

Occupational Safety and Health Administration: *OSHA standards.* Washington, DC: Author, 1970.

Pabst MK, Scherubel JC, and Minnick AF: The impact of computerized documentation on nurses' use of time. *Computers in Nursing* 14 (1), 25-30, 1996.

Pearson L: Annual update of how each state stands on legislative issues affecting advanced nursing practice. *The Nurse Practitioner* 23 (1): 14-16, 19, 1998.

Pillitteri A: *Maternal and child health nursing.* Philadelphia: J. B. Lippincott, 1996.

Potter P and Perry A: *Basic nursing: Theory and practice.* 3rd ed. St. Louis, MO: C. V. Mosby, 1995.

Powers M: Legal protections of confidential medical information and the need for anti-discrimination laws. In *AIDS, women, and the next generation,* R Faden, G Geller, and M Powers, eds. New York: Oxford University Press, 1991, pp. 221-255.

Price PJ: Parents' perceptions of the meaning of quality nursing care. *Advances in Nursing Science* 16 (1): 33-41, 1993.

Pruett JJ: Chronic substandard staffing and the nurse's liability. *Critical Care Nurse* 13 (4): 88-93, 1993.

Quigley FM: Standards of care: Part I. *Focus Critical Care* 18 (5): 390-391, 1991a.

Quigley FM: Standards of care: Part II. *Focus Critical Care* 18 (6): 474-475, 1991b.

Reed K: Computerization of health care information: More automation, less privacy. *Journal of Health and Hospital Law* 27 (12): 353-368, 1994.

Rhodes AM: The need for security with computerized records. *MCN: American Journal of Maternal Child Nursing* 20: 299, 1995.

Rini AG: Confidentiality. In *NGNA core curriculum for gerontological advanced practice nurses,* AS Luggen, SS Travis, and SE Meiner, eds. Thousand Oaks, CA: Sage, 1998.

Robinson D, Anderson M, and Erpenbeck P: Telephone advice: New solutions for old problems. *The Nurse Practitioner* 22 (3): 179-190, 1997.

Rosenblatt RE, Law SA, and Rosenbaum S: *Law and the American health care system.* Westbury, NY: Foundation Press, 1997.

Rustia JG and Bartek JK: Managed care credentialing of advanced practice nurses. *The Nurse Practitioner* 22 (9): 90, 92, 99-100, 102-103, 1997.

Safriet E: Health care dollars and regulatory sense: The role of advanced practice nursing. *Yale Journal of Regulation* 9: 479, 1992.

Schwartz AE: *Delegating authority.* New York: Barrons Educational System, 1992.

Scott M and Packard K: *Telephone assessment with protocols for nursing practice.* Philadelphia: W. B. Saunders, 1990.

Sebas M: Developing a collaborative practice agreement for the primary care setting. *The Nurse Practitioner* 19: 49-51, 1994.

Sheehan J and Sullivan GH: Liability issues in development, implementation, and documentation of critical pathways. In *Planning, implementing, and evaluating critical pathways: A guide for health care survival into the 21st century,* PC Dykes and K Wheeler, eds. New York: Springer, 1997.

Shortliffe E, Tang P, Amatayakul M, Cottington E, Jencks S, Martin A, MacDonald R, Morris T, and Nobel J: Future vision and dissemination of computer-based patient records. In *Aspects of computer-based patient records,* M Ball and M Collen, eds. New York: Springer-Verlag, 1992.

Siegrist L, Dettor R, and Stocks B: The PIE system: Planning and documentation of nursing care. *Quality Review Bulletin* 11 (6): 186-189, 1985.

Smeltzer C: The art of negotiation: An everyday experience. *Journal of Nursing Administration* 21: 23-30, 1991.

Soreff S and McDuffee M (Eds.): *Documentation survival handbook for psychiatrists and other mental health professionals.* Seattle, WA: Hogrefe & Huber, 1993.

Springhouse: *Mastering documentation.* Springhouse, PA: Springhouse Corporation, 1995.

Springhouse: *Tips and time savers for home health nurses.* Springhouse, PA: Springhouse Corporation, 1997.

Stuart GW and Laraia MT: *Principles and practice of psychiatric nursing.* 6th ed. St. Louis, MO: C. V. Mosby, 1997.

Tadych R: *Collaborative practice agreement checklist* [brochure]. Jefferson City, MO: Missouri State Board of Nursing, 1997.

Tammelleo AD: Charting by exception: There are perils. *RN* 57 (10): 71-72, 1994.

Thacker SB, Stroup DF, Parrish RG, and Anderson HA: Surveillance in environmental public health: Issues, systems, and sources. *American Journal of Public Health* 86 (5): 633-638, 1996.

Tracy N, Hoffman C, Barrows R, Clayton P, and Wald J: Privacy protection: Paper or computer records? *Behavioral Healthcare Tomorrow* 5 (1): 38-44, 1996.

Trandel-Korenchuk DM and Trandel-Korenchuk K: *Nursing and the law.* 5th ed. Gaithersburg, MD: Aspen, 1997.

U.S. Department of Health and Human Services: *Minimizing restraints in nursing homes: A guide to action.* Washington, DC: Author, 1992.

U.S. Department of Health and Human Services: *Treatment of pressure ulcers: Clinical practice guidelines.* Rockville, MD: Agency for Health Care Policy and Research, 1996.

Urden LD, Davie JK, and Thelan LA: *Essentials of critical care nursing.* St. Louis, MO: C. V. Mosby, 1992.

Waegemann CP: The future role of patient cards [abstract]. In *Toward an electronic patient record '98.* Newton, MA: Medical Records Institute, 1998a.

Waegemann CP: Overview of standards developments [abstract]. In *Toward an electronic patient record '98.* Newton, MA: Medical Records Institute, 1998b.

Waller AA: Appendix B: Legal aspects of computer-based patient records and record systems. In *The computer-based patient record: An essential technology for health care,* R Dick and E Steen, eds. Washington, DC: National Academy Press, 1991.

Waller AA and Darrah JM: Legal requirements for computer security: Electronic medical records and data interchange. *Behavioral Healthcare Tomorrow* 5 (1): 45-47, 1996.

Weber J and Kelley J: *Health assessment in nursing.* Philadelphia: Lippincott-Raven, 1998.

Weissenstein E: Providers dispute patient privacy bill. *Modern Healthcare* 26 (23): 32, 1996.

Wenner AR: Physicians academy [abstract]. In *Toward an electronic patient record '98.* Newton, MA: Medical Records Institute, 1998.

West CD: Pediatric nomogram. In *Nelson textbook of pediatrics,* 14th ed., RE Behrman and VS Vaughan, eds. Philadelphia: W. B. Saunders, 1992.

Westin AF: *Privacy and freedom.* New York: Atheneum, 1967.

Wiger DE: *The clinical documentation sourcebook: A comprehensive collection of mental health practice forms, handouts, and records.* New York: John Wiley, 1997.

Wong DL: *Wong and Whaley's clinical manual of pediatric nursing.* 4th ed. St. Louis, MO: C. V. Mosby, 1996.

Woody RH: *Legally safe mental health practice.* Madison, CT: Psychosocial Press, 1997.

Yocke JM and Donner TA: Floating out of the ICU: The ethical dilemmas. II. The case analysis. *Dimensions of Critical Care Nursing* 11 (2): 105-107, 1992.

Younger P, Conner C, Cartwright K, and Kole S: *Legal answer book for managed care.* Gaithersburg, MD: Aspen, 1995.

LEGAL CASE REFERENCES

Atkinson v. Traetta, 359 N.Y.S. 2d 120, 1974.

Batra v. Board of Regents of University of Nebraska, 79 F3d 717, 1996.

Bigbee v. Pacific Telephone and Telegraph Co., 665 P. 2d 947, Calif., 1983.

Board of Curators of the University of Missouri v. Horowitz, 435 U.S. 78, 98 W. Ct. 948, 1978.

Buckley v. Hospital Corporation of America, 758 F. 2d 1525, 11th Cir., 1985.

Darling v. Charleston Community Memorial Hospital, 211 N.E. 2d 253, Ill., 1965.

Derdiarian v. Felix Contracting Corp., 414 N.E. 2d, 666, 670, N.Y., 1980.

Edwards v. Brandywine Hospital, 652 A. 2d 1382, Pa. Sup., 1995.

Federal Register, V56187, p. 48825, September 26, 1991.

Hillis v. Stephen F. Austin State University, 665 Fed. 2d 547, 1982.

In re Westchester County Medical Center, No. 91-504-2, Decision No. CR 191, Department of Health and Human Services, Departmental Appeals Board, Civil Remedies Division, April 20, 1992.

McIntosh v. Borough of Manhattan Community College, 78 App. Div., 2d 839, 433, N.Y.S. 2d 446, 1980.

Missouri Revised Statutes, Section 335.016, 1995.

Missouri Statutes, Section 334.194, RS Mo., 1995.

Nassau County, Florida v. Arline, 480 U.S. 273, 1987.

New Mexico Statutes Annotated, Chapter 61, 1992.

Norfolk Protestant Hospital v. Plunket, 173 S.E. 363, Va., 1934.

Phillips v. Oconee Memorial Hospital, 290 S.C., 192, 348 S.E. 2d 836, S.C., 1986.

Regents of the University of Michigan v. Ewing, 88 L.Ed. 2d 523, 101 S. Ct. 507, 1985.

Ross v. Pennsylvania State University, 445 F. Supp. 147, 1978.

Schuler v. University of Minnesota, 788 F2d 510, 1986.

Schlussler v. Independent School District No. 200 et al., Case No. MM89-14V, Minnesota Case Reports, Minn., 1989.

Sermchief v. Gonzales, 660 S.W. 2d 683, Missouri en Banc, 1983.

State ex rel Keeney v. Ayres, 109 Montana 547, 92 P2d 306, 1939.

State ex rel Richardson v. Board of Regents, 70 Nevada 144, 261 P2d 515, 1953.

Thompson v. Nason Hospital, 591 A.2d 703, Pa., 1991.

Wallace v. Veterans Administration, 683 F. Supp. 758, D. Kan., 1988.

Yucker v. University of Florida, 602 So2d 557, 1992.

Zumwalt v. Trustees of California State Colleges, 33 Cal. App. 3d 655, 109 Cal. Rptr. 344, 1973.

GLOSSARY

ACOG: American College of Obstetricians and Gynecologists

Adequate staffing: Sufficient numbers of qualified staff in health care institutions to meet accreditation standards

Administrative agency: An arm of the government that administers or carries out legislative enactments; may be federal, state, or local

Admission requirements: Statements of requirements that students must fulfill before being allowed admission to a school or an institution

Admitting privileges: Rights granted by individual health care institutions that allow physicians and other independent practitioners, including advanced practice nurses, the ability to admit patients to the facilities

Advanced directives: The various methods used by competent adults to indicate their choices in health care treatment decisions including, but are not limited to, express verbal communications, living wills, durable powers of attorney, and trust agreements

Advanced nursing practice: Refers to CNS, NP, CRNA, and CNM

Advanced practice nurse: A registered nurse with specialized education, experience, and skill who is authorized to perform acts of prevention, medical diagnosis, and the prescription of medical, therapeutic, or corrective measures as determined by regulations approved by the individual state board of nursing

Affidavit: Voluntary written statement made or taken under oath before an officer of the court or a notary public; usually a sworn statement of facts

Age of majority: Statutory or legal age of adulthood, generally 18 years

Agency personnel: Nurses who are hired by health care institutions to work a specific shift and who are not full- or part-time workers of the institution but, rather, employees of agencies that provide temporary help

Agency policy: Written communications that set the standard of care for a given health care agency

Agent: The person authorized by another to act for him or her

Allegation: A statement, charge, or assertion that a person expects to be able to prove to others

Alteration of records: Entries added to a patient record necessary to ensure a truthful and accurate report; can be either minor (e.g., spelling) or substantive (e.g., omitted nurses notes, incorrect orders, incorrect laboratory data)

ANA: American Nurses Association

ANCC: American Nurses Credentialing Center (of ANA)

ANP: Advanced nursing practice

AORN: Association of Operating Room Nurses

APN: Advanced practice nurse

Appeal: A legal proceeding in which a higher court is asked to reverse or correct the decision of a lower court

AWHONN: Association of Women's Health, Obstetric, and Neonatal Nurses (formerly known as Nurses Association of the American Academy of Obstetricians and Gynecologists [NAACOG])

Battery: Intentional and wrongful physical contact with a person without consent

Breach: Failure of performance by a person with a legal duty owed to someone

Breach of duty: Deviation from standard of care owed to another

CBAPR: Computer-based accessible patient record

CBR: Computer-based patient record

Certification: Programs sponsored by private, nongovernmental, professional organizations or agencies that recognize the attainment of advanced, specialized knowledge and skills beyond what is necessary for safe practice

Certified nurse midwife: Training at the master's degree level in nursing

Certified nursing specialist (or clinical nurse specialist): A registered nurse with specialized education, experience, and skill who is authorized to teach, direct, and apply advanced nursing knowledge in a clinical setting

CHHR: Clinical home health record

Civil law: Used to distinguish that part of the law concerned with noncriminal matters

CMIT: Current medical information and terminology

CNM: Certified nurse midwife

CNS: Certified nursing specialist; clinical nurse specialist

Collaborative practice: Joint practice arrangement with one or more other health care providers

Common law: Law consisting of broad and comprehensive principles; the body of law that develops through judicial decisions

Complaint: A petition or an application in writing to the court or judge stating the facts and circumstances relied on as a cause for judicial action and containing a formal request for relief

Consent: A voluntary action by which an individual agrees to allow someone else to do something; may be oral, written, or implied based on the circumstances

Continuing treatment doctrine: Extended time to enter medical malpractice action when the course of treatment following wrongful acts or omissions continues; must be related to the original condition or complaint

Counterclaim: An individual cause of action made by a defendant against the plaintiff, the purpose of which is to oppose or deduct from the plaintiff's claim

CPA: Collaborative practice agreement

CPT: Current procedural terminology

Credentials: Proof of qualifications stating that an individual or organization has met certain standards (e.g., licensure, certification)

CRNA: Certified registered nurse anesthetist

Diagnosis-related groups: Pertaining to the Medicare and Medicaid system for reimbursement of charges to private or public health care providers

Discovery: The pretrial devices that can be used by one party to obtain facts and information about the case from the other party to assist in the preparation for trial

Discovery rule: The limitation statute in malpractice cases that does not begin to accrue until the date of discovery of the malpractice

DRGs: Diagnosis-related groups

DSM-IV: *Diagnostic and Statistical Manual of Mental Disorders* (fourth edition) of the American Psychiatric Association

Due process: Law in its regular course of administration through courts of justice

Duty: Legal or moral obligation that one has to conform to a legal standard of reasonable conduct in light of apparent risk

Ethics: Science relating to moral actions and moral values; rules of conduct recognized in respect to a particular class of human actions

Evidence: All factual matters that are presented for investigation at judicial trial

Expert witness: A witness having special knowledge of the subject about which he or she is to testify; witness whose knowledge generally must be such that it is not normally possessed by the average person; contrasting with lay witness

Expressed consent: Written or oral permission to perform an act

Failure to warn: A newer area of potential liability for nurses involving the responsibility to warn potential victims of violent acts that have been threatened by others; requires a thorough understanding of the laws of confidentiality

False imprisonment: The unjustified detention or confinement of a person without legal warrant; an intentional tort

Fire wall: Security access control for computer systems with network or multistation work settings; limit of access to computer information

Float personnel: Health care employees who are required to rotate to other than their usual units of practice during times of staffing shortage in other areas

Fraudulent concealment doctrine: Hiding or suppression of a material fact or circumstance that the party is legally or morally bound to disclose

Good Samaritan laws: Individual state legislative enactments passed to encourage health care providers and citizens trained in first aid to deliver needed medical care at accident sites and roadside emergencies without unnecessary fear of incurring criminal or civil liability

HCFA: Health Care Financing Administration

Health Care Financing Administration: Oversees long-term care agencies

HHCC: Home health care classification

ICD: International classification of diseases

ICHPPC: International classification of health problems in primary care

ICNP: International classification of nursing practice

Implied consent: Permission inferred by the patient's actions (e.g., head nodding, holding out an arm for a blood draw) or legally presumed (e.g., emergency consent)

Incident form: Any variation, situation, or unusual occurrence in health care, mandated by JCAHO, to be used for quality improvement and patient review and evaluation of care; not always discoverable in lawsuits

Incision: Intentional cut through intact tissue

INIC: Iowa nursing intervention classification

JCAHO: Joint Commission on Accreditation of Healthcare Organizations

Joint Commission on Accreditation of Healthcare Organizations: Voluntary group of health care professionals that inspects and scores health care facilities on standards of operation

Judgment: Determination of a court of competent jurisdiction to matters submitted to the court; a final determination of the rights of the parties to an action

KONA: New standard markup language similar to that used on the Internet to ease the creation and exchange of computer-based patient records

Liability: Responsibility for personal conduct; an obligation or duty to be performed

Licensure: A right granted that gives licensees permission to do something that they could not legally do without such permission; as a personal right, generally nontransferable and not assignable

Malfeasance: Wrongdoing; ill conduct; commission of some act that is unlawful

Malpractice: Professional misconduct or unreasonable lack of skill; failure of one rendering professional services to exercise the degree of skill and learning commonly applied under all circumstances in the community by the average prudent and reputable member of the profession, with the result of injury (loss or damage) to the recipient of those services

MDS: Minimum Data Set

Minimum Data Set: Recording format required in long-term care facilities

NAACOG: Nurses Association of the American Academy of Obstetricians and Gynecologists (former name of organization now named AWHONN)

NANDA: North American Nursing Diagnosis Association

NCS: Nursing classification system

NCSBN: National Council of State Boards of Nursing

Negligence: Failure to use such care as a reasonably prudent and careful person would use under similar circumstances

NLN: National League of Nursing

North American Nursing Diagnosis Association: Founding organization of terminology related to nursing diagnosis

NPA: Nurse Practice Act

NP: Nurse practitioner

Nurse Practice Act: Statutory enactment that defines the practice of nursing and gives guidance with scope of practice issues; passes on a state-to-state basis

Nurse practitioner: An advanced practice nurse with a specialty field

Occupational health nurse: Nursing at business or work settings (e.g., industrial setting)

Occupational Safety and Health Administration: Oversees the healthful and safe working conditions in the workplace

OHN: Occupational health nurse

OSHA: Occupational Safety and Health Administration

Personal liability: Responsibility and accountability for one's own actions

PIE: Problem-intervention-evaluation format for documenting nursing care

Plaintiff: Party bringing a civil lawsuit that seeks damages or other relief; at trial, the injured party or representative thereof

Policies and procedures: Part of risk management, the written documents that set standards of care for a given health care institution

POMR: Problem-oriented medical record

Prescriptive privileges (authority): The legal right to determine pharmaco-therapeutic management for patients

Protocols: Statements written and used by nurses in expanded roles that outline and authorize particular practice activities

Public law: The branch of law concerned with the state in its political capacity

READ Codes: Controlled medical vocabulary produced during the Clinical Terms Projects with the involvement of more than 2,000 health care professionals from all U.K. specialties

Reasonable or prudent patient standard: Test of informed consent based on the needs of what a prudent person in the patient's position would deem material about the disclosure of risks and benefits of a proposed treatment; may be divided into objective patient standard and subjective patient standard

Release: Signed statement relinquishing a right or claim against another person, usually for valuable consideration; accompanies a settlement to prevent a future lawsuit on the same issues or occurrence

Respondeat superior: Latin term meaning "Let the master answer," meaning that the employer is liable in certain cases for the wrongful acts of the employee; also called master-servant or vicarious liability

Restraints: Chemical, mechanical, or physical measures that prevent patient freedom

Scope of practice: The boundaries and limitations placed on a discipline's professional practice by legislative, legal, and professional groups

SNOMED: Systemized nomenclature of human and veterinary medicine

SOAP: Charting format that follows a pattern of information—subjective, objective, assessment, and plan

SOAPE: Charting format that follows a pattern of information—subjective, objective, assessment, plan, and evaluation

SOAPIER: Charting format that follows a pattern of information—subjective, objective, assessment, plan, evaluation, and revision

Standards of care: The degree of care that a reasonably prudent person should exercise in the same or similar circumstances; in malpractice cases, applied to measure the competence of the professional

Standards of practice: Minimal levels of accepted performance by members of a professional discipline

Statute: A particular law enacted and established by the will of the legislative department of government

Statutory laws: Rules and regulations (also called statutes) created by legislative bodies such as Congress, state houses, and city councils

Suicide prevention: An obligation of nurses to protect patients from self-harm

Tort: A private or civil wrong or injury, usually including a violation of a duty

Triage: To sort, classify, and/or choose for immediate or delayed action

UAP: Unlicenced assistive personnel

UCDS: Uniform clinical data set

UMLS: Unified medical language system

Unlicenced assistive personnel: Persons employed in health care settings to augment patient care; persons without licensure under an NPA

UNLS: Unified Nursing Language System

Values: Personal beliefs about the truths and worth of thoughts, objects, or behavior; motives and attitudes; and the relationship of these motives and attitudes to the good of the person

Vicarious liability: The liability of the employer for the acts of an employee

Voir dire: Latin term for the process of selecting a jury; the process of determining the qualifications of an expert witness during deposition or trial

Wound: Injury to tissue by intent or accident

Wound, clean: No foreign matter present; healing by first intention after closure

Wound, clean contaminated: Classification of surgical incision that has had a nonsterile item near or in a sterile field

Wound, contaminated: Incision invaded by nonsterile and bacteria-containing items

Wound, dirty: Foreign bodies and microorganisms with potential for infection

Wound, infected: Invasion of the incision by pathogenic microorganisms and the reaction of tissues to their presence

Index

AUTHOR AND CONTRIBUTORS

Author:

Sue E. Meiner, EdD, RN, CS, GNP, is a gerontological advanced practice nurse, multidisciplinary gerontologist, research patient coordinator, and project director of a National Institute of Health/National Institute of Aging grant at Washington University Medical School, Division of Geriatrics/Gerontology, in St. Louis, Missouri. She holds the academic rank of associate professor at the Jewish Hospital College of Nursing and Allied Health. She has continued to practice patient-centered nursing while conducting research, publishing articles and books, and presenting workshops and seminars in local, regional, and national venues. Her community service experience includes holding an elected office for 5 years in a suburb of St. Louis. She has been involved in legal nurse consulting and has served as an expert witness in litigation for plaintiff and defense claims. Her work includes medical record review and analysis, deposition reviews, literature research and evaluation, preparing reports and affidavits, being deposed, and giving testimony during trial appearances. The Missouri State Board of Nursing recognizes her as an advanced practice nurse. She has attained dual certification from the American Nurses Credentialing Center of the American Nurses Association as a gerontological clinical nurse specialist and as a gerontological nurse practitioner.

Contributors:

Marilee Kuhrik, PhD, RN, and **Nancy Kuhrik,** PhD, RN, each completed more than 30 years of service with the Barnes-Jewish Hospital. As associate professors with the Jewish Hospital College of Nursing and Allied Health, the two sisters were active in clinical instruction, student activities, publishing in nursing journals and books, and community and alumni projects. Recently, they relocated to Colorado to continue their teaching careers as associate professors at Colorado Mountain College, Roaring Fork Campus, Glenwood Springs.

Robyn Levy, MSN, CS, ANP, has provided nursing service in the Barnes-Jewish Hospital Health Care System for more than 20 years. She began in nursing service as a staff nurse. Following completion of advanced degrees, she transferred to the Jewish Hospital College of Nursing and Allied Health. She holds certification as an adult nurse practitioner. Although she is an active adult nurse practitioner, she continues as an assistant professor with responsibilities for coordinating the nurse practitioner master's program.

Elizabeth C. Mueth, MLS, AHIP, has been a librarian for the past 17 years. She is an active member and past president of the St. Louis Medical Librarians. She has held certification from the Medical Librarians Association for 13 years. As an assistant professor with the Jewish Hospital College of Nursing and Allied Health, she is responsible for teaching all computer-based classes. She also serves as the World Wide Web master for the college. Her current involvement is in development of a smart classroom and distance learning center.

Alice G. Rini, JD, MSN, RN, after many years in nursing and nursing education, completed studies in law and earned a juris doctorate. She currently is a practicing attorney in northern Kentucky while she continues teaching as an associate professor of law at Northern Kentucky University.

Linda Steele, PhD, RN, CS, ANP, is an associate professor in the Adult Health College of Nursing and Health Professions at the University of North Carolina at Charlotte. She has a nursing career that extends more than 25 years and is certified as an adult nurse practitioner. While serving as an active health care provider, she continues to teach nursing students at the baccalaureate and master's levels.

Linda L. Zinser-Eagle, BSN, RN, has been associated with the Barnes-Jewish Hospital since 1971. She practiced perioperative nursing before becoming an educator in perioperative nursing. Since 1978, her progressive responsibilities have included all areas of perioperative nursing practice and instruction to nurses and ancillary operating room technicians. Her current position is that of a perioperative educator.